Moving
from the
Inside Out

Moving from the Inside Out

7 **Principles** *for* Ease *and* Mastery *in* Movement

A Feldenkrais Approach

LESLEY McLENNAN AND JULIE PECK

North Atlantic Books
Berkeley, California

Somatic Resources
San Diego, California

Published by
North Atlantic Books   and   Somatic Resources
Berkeley, California   San Diego, California

Cover design by Howie Severson
Book design by Happenstance Type-O-Rama
Cover photo © gettyimages.com/Henrik Sorensen
Interior photos/illustrations © Lesley McLennan, Sharon Felschow, Shutterstock

Feldenkrais®, Feldenkrais Method®, Functional Integration®, Awareness Through Movement®, and Guild Certified Feldenkrais Practitioner® are service marks of the Feldenkrais Guild® of North America.

Printed in Canada

Moving from the Inside Out: 7 Principles for Ease and Mastery in Movement is sponsored and published by the Society for the Study of Native Arts and Sciences (dba North Atlantic Books), an educational nonprofit based in Berkeley, California, that collaborates with partners to develop cross-cultural perspectives, nurture holistic views of art, science, the humanities, and healing, and seed personal and global transformation by publishing work on the relationship of body, spirit, and nature.

North Atlantic Books' publications are available through most bookstores. For further information, visit our website at www.northatlanticbooks.com or call 800-733-3000.

MEDICAL DISCLAIMER: The following information is intended for general information purposes only. Individuals should always see their health care provider before administering any suggestions made in this book. Any application of the material set forth in the following pages is at the reader's discretion and is his or her sole responsibility.

Library of Congress Cataloging-in-Publication Data

Names: McLennan, Lesley, 1958- author. | Peck, Julie, 1956– author. |
    Society for the Study of Native Arts and Sciences, sponsoring body.
Title: Moving from the inside out : 7 principles for ease and mastery in
    movement / Lesley McLennan & Julie Peck.
Description: Berkeley, California : North Atlantic Books ; San Diego,
    California : Somatic Resources, [2020] | "[S]ponsored and published by
    the Society for the Study of Native Arts and Sciences." | Includes
    bibliographical references and index.
Identifiers: LCCN 2019053785 | ISBN 9781623175085 (paperback) | ISBN
    9781623175092 (epub)
Subjects: LCSH: Feldenkrais method. | Movement therapy.
Classification: LCC RC489.F44 M35 2020 | DDC 616.89/165—dc23
LC record available at https://lccn.loc.gov/2019053785

1 2 3 4 5 6 7 8 9 MARQUIS 24 23 22 21 20

CONTENTS

LIST OF ILLUSTRATIONS

LIST OF TIYS

STARTING POINTS

HOW MIGHT A TIGHT tummy lead to voice loss?

- What do swinging an axe and a baby's first means of propulsion have in common?
- How can a bathroom scale test your skeletal alignment?
- What can we learn from giraffes about balance?
- And—how can you use this information to live a better life?

This book is about movement. That is synonymous with saying this book is about life. From the first twitch in the womb to the last dying flicker of the nervous system, our lives are movement. In all its diverse aspects—as sensation, thought, action, or emotion—movement is life.

Most often we focus on the results of our actions, rarely noticing how we move. Our attention is drawn to our patterns and habits of movement only when we have pain or dysfunction, or when we wish to learn a new skill or to perform at an elite level.

In the following pages we use seven organizing principles to ignite curiosity in our own, and others', movements. This is not a text about anatomical or physiological details. It presents perspectives that can augment insights from coaches, therapists, teachers, or research. We all need experts in our lives who can provide pointers and shortcuts to our desired outcomes, but the seven principles are for those nonurgent times, when, through our own explorations, we can lay foundations to become expert in our own patterns.

The Power of Principles

A long, long time ago, humans discovered that a key to understanding complexity was to search for underlying similarities: patterns that connect and principles that explain. Some principles (or laws) are so foundational that we begin teaching them as children's tales. We are told how Archimedes discovered the principle of buoyancy by stepping into a bathtub—famously solving the question of a fraudulent gold crown—and how Newton, hit by a falling apple, discovered the law of gravity, thus explaining the moon's rotation around Earth.

A good principle helps us discover "aha" moments by erasing boundaries that exist in our thinking but not in the natural world. Interesting connections appear, giving us novel solutions. It is now commonplace to talk about the problems of intellectually separating mind and body—yet this separation has ruled Western thinking for centuries. It stimulated important discoveries but has also led to unhelpful oversights. Similarly in this book we will sometimes use conceptual distinctions between thinking, sensing, and feeling to help explore ideas; the intention is not to isolate or separate, but to reintegrate these components in our image of movement.

If the principles are robust, they will hold true across culture, race, and even species. They will be applicable in a range of contexts including therapy, performance, martial arts, self-development, and working with animals. You will be able to actively test them in your field of interest as you read further.

Our seven organizing principles of movement have no hierarchical order. They interconnect, and ultimately are designed to be a bridge from the abstract world of theory to the concrete world of actions. They should be lightly held, playfully explored, and mined for applications.

The Power of Distinctions

Distinctions separate by defining differences, but they can also unify by unearthing similarity or interconnections commonly overlooked. With ever-finer distinctions we gain ever-finer understanding and control, because distinctions enable us to learn.

In regular conversation, **movement** refers to something we can see—a physical shift in shape or position—whether it is as subtle as a twitch of the eyelid or as gross as a leap through space. We commonly categorize movement as physical activity, thinking as mental activity, and sensing and feeling as emotional activities. Yet in this book we are suggesting that movement is an integration of thinking, sensing, and feeling with action in such a way that a change in one will change the whole. The components may be distinct, but they are not separable in a functioning human.

There will be many opportunities in the coming chapters to consider why this is important in practical terms. For now, let's clarify the distinctions between two components that are easily confused.

Sensing pertains to information from the receptors of our nervous system—the receptors bring us information from both our external and internal environments. We can sense temperature, pressure, light, color, vibrations, position, and so on. When we describe sensory experience, we will use words that describe texture, weight, volume, maybe intervals or intensity. Even though it is common to say we "feel" these distinctions, these are our sensations, not our feelings.

Feelings are constructed from sensation, that is, internal sensory information from our interoceptors. Commonly we distinguish between feelings that we regard as physiological (tired, hungry, jittery) versus emotional (happy, disgusted, enamored), but in the context of movement we are using "feelings" to represent both.

Sensing gives us very important information on our internal and external environment. We can usually find objective consensus for sensory information; that is, we can agree on what is lighter or heavier, less or more salty, and so on. Feelings are more subjective, less available to consensus, but not less important. Internal sensation is corralled into the primary division of feelings—pleasant or unpleasant—so swiftly that our comparatively slow cognitive processes (our thinking) rarely notice the inception of feeling—the beginning of every emotion we experience.

Both sensing and feeling are enormously important to how we experience and move in the world.

Human movements (or those of any other animal) are shaped as much by the external environment as by all the internal factors. Our social, cultural, and physical environments are an inseparable part of how we develop and move through the world, and they always need to be considered when improving, changing, or developing movement.

The Power of Stories

Stories bridge theory and practice. From parables to case studies, stories help clarify meaning, stimulate memory, and provide clues for use. What starts as a grand statement or an abstract concept can expand into an actionable idea through the power of stories. We'll be using many stories throughout this book to illustrate concepts. They have been drawn from our own experiences, and those of our colleagues and teachers. Names and identifying details have, of course, been changed.

We have made up only one story, our first. It is an adaptation of an old parable, used to illustrate some foundational themes of this book.

A Parable of Perspectives

Moving with ease and mastery is one of the greatest pleasures of life. Yet from a young age we encounter rules, constraints, and dogmas that limit our choices. Once we have internalized rules and dogmas, it is difficult to even recognize them. Every now and then we need to play with new perspectives, which is where the story of the blind men and the elephant comes in.

Once upon a time, an elephant appeared in a village. Elephants were unknown in the region, and the citizens were mystified. They couldn't believe their eyes, so they sent for the village elders—seven blind men—to explain this new phenomenon.

Each one laid his hands on a different part of the elephant, investigating his area in detail and then began to speak. The blind man standing at the side of the elephant found the beast was rather like a wall. The one at the ear felt the wall but found the delicate flapping lobe of greater import, and he opined the beast was rather like a fan. The blind man who explored the trunk explained that the beast was rather like a snake. For tail and leg and tusk, each of the elders chose something familiar to explain the beast.

The seventh blind man, who was a little more adventurous than his colleagues, shimmied up the tree that shaded the elephant, and slowly he inched out on an overhanging branch, hoping the creature might now be under him. To his delight, it was, so he gently eased himself onto the broad back of the elephant.

Meanwhile, at ground level, things were getting heated. Each wise man spoke with eloquence and vehemence, wanting to convince the others of his own perspective. As often happens when opinions differ, a fight broke out. That was enough for the elephant, and off it went down the road with the adventurous blind man scrambling to stay seated astride its shoulders while the villagers scattered in fear.

Ahh, what a privileged seat. The seventh blind man could feel the whole elephant galvanize into action. He could sense skin, muscle, and bone and oh so much more. The great head led the forward direction as the shoulders and spine tilted and turned beneath him. The legs moved in a rhythm contrapuntal to the breathtaking ribs. He could sense through subtle changes that just as his own fright was diminishing, so too was the elephant's. Gradually man and beast settled into a pleasurable rhythmic partnership. And that is where he found his own description—not just for the elephant, but for the uniting of elephant and man in movement. "We," thought the blind man, "are rather like a dance."

When the seventh blind man was rescued safely from the back of the creature, he stood motionless on the ground for a few moments, noticing that after the adventure he felt very, very different.

His curiosity had placed him in a unique position. The six other elders had worked with their hands and their heads as they usually did, and found one strong and static perspective each, as they usually did. His was the novel experience, where those habits were no longer helpful.

He was thrust into a larger arena of awareness than he had ever used before, where he needed to think, move, sense, and feel differently. This was both a bigger and a simpler way of knowing the world than he had ever imagined, and he dedicated the rest of his life to it.

From Parable to Wonder

The parable of the six blind men and the elephant has a very long history. It first appeared more than two millennia ago and has been retold many times since. Obviously humans have always needed a reminder of our tendency to fixate on single perspectives, when many more are available and important.

We've cheekily added a seventh man to the story, also blind, also taking only one position on the elephant from which to form his opinion. But from this position on the beast's back, he can experience the elephant using more of his body and all his senses, inside and out. He can feel skin, flesh, and bone, and he can also feel rhythm and response, not just in the animal but in himself as well.

The seventh man's dedication is ours too—dedication to the wonder of knowing ourselves, other people, and the world around us, in the most direct manner possible, through movement.

Seven Organizing Principles of Movement

The idea behind the organizing principles (OPs) is to understand patterns that are, or would be, innate to us if our nervous systems developed without internal or external disruption.

Consider these as the three criteria for well-organized movement:

- Is it effective? Does it fulfill your intentions?
- Is it efficient? Is it the best use of your individual structure and current abilities?
- Is it sustainable and sustaining—intellectually, emotionally, physically, and spiritually?

Why **organizing** principles? We have mentioned "organizing" several times in this book already. It may not be a word you usually connect with movement. Organizing (and organization) in general use indicates bringing order to chaos by imposing systems. In movement, the source of order is not imposed but innate: our own nervous systems bring order to the chaos of incoming and outgoing signals that movement depends on. The organization of movement grows and matures with the developing nervous system. Other than physical and neurological damage, the greatest disruptions of our innate organization come from imposed social and individual expectations.

So here are the principles we will discuss in much greater depth in the following chapters:

OP1. Balance is dynamic
All movement requires a dynamic balance between stability and instability.

OP2. Skeletal alignment liberates movement
When the skeleton is aligned for support, large muscles are freed for action and movement becomes light and powerful.

OP3. Progress to upright is cyclical
Evolving to stand upright with a 360-degree view of the world is a sequential progression that is revisited with each major movement challenge.

OP4. Qualities refine self-direction
Attention to quality of movement creates an internal reference system for exploring movement, recognizing unconscious habits, and learning new ways to move.

OP5. Head guides and pelvis drives
Efficient movement requires a head that is free to orient us, connected by an adaptable spine to the power generated at the pelvis.

OP6. Power is central and precision peripheral
Strength and force come from the center, while direction and accuracy come from the extremities.

OP7. Pressure organizes
The demands of internal or external pressure create and test our ability to respond with well-organized movement.

The Presence of Absence

The principles are a way to recognize both the patterns and potentials in our movement. Stimulating or restoring an absent potential has immense therapeutic value and will often be where the principles are most usefully applied. Yet noticing absence—knowing what we don't know, or seeing what is missing—is easier said than done.

There are two aspects to consider regarding absence. First, we are quicker to notice the presence of struggle, pain, or discomfort than its absence. When you are experiencing difficulties and then they disappear, you might think it would be immediately obvious. More commonly it can be days, weeks, or months before remembering: "Oh, I used to get a pain when I did this—I wonder when that changed?" By the time we notice the absence, we cannot remember exactly what made the difference, so we do not build on our best strategies for change. Because ease, grace, and pleasure occur in the absence of struggle, pain, and discomfort, regularly searching for these three delights helps us notice change—and our role in it—more efficiently.

The second aspect is an absence in our image of movement. We need an idea that something is possible, or even exists, before we search for it. For example, most things you can do with your fingers you can also do with your toes (interlace them, cross them, type with them), but few of us have ever explored this potential because we never thought to do so—the idea was absent in our image of toe movements. We all have these absences or blind spots, some common, some unique, but each hiding a piece of our potential. They are hard to see in ourselves or to illuminate for others; to identify them we must both recognize that they could exist and observe from multiple angles in case they do. In this book we explain concepts, tell stories, share images, and recommend experiments—all to help you glimpse these gaps. Reading with an open mind, one that can shift perspectives and bring curiosity before judgment, will also help you identify absence and opportunity. With the right attitude, discovering absences becomes an exciting arrow to imminent potential.

Neuroplasticity

Underlying all the principles is an acknowledgment that change is a constant in our lives, not an intermittent event. Compelling evidence of neuroplastic change has inspired great excitement and research in the past few decades, debunking old beliefs about the fixed nature of a mature human nervous system. Put simply, neuroplasticity is the ability for your brain to make new connections between neurons. New connections, or rewiring, means abilities can develop, expand, or be recovered. New connections form when an activity is novel, we give it our attention, we repeat it, and it is pleasurable. Like all simple explanations, this quick sketch leaves out many details and permutations.

You don't need to understand neuroplasticity to get value from this book. However, in those moments when change is slow, when abilities seem irretrievable or beyond us, it may comfort you to know that science supports our potential to either recover abilities or develop new ones if we choose strategies that best suit our nervous system—that is, strategies that include novelty, attention, repetition with variation, and pleasure.

Neuroplasticity is a property of our brains that does not discriminate good from bad. We are all capable of repeating novel activities, with attention and with elevated emotions, that will have a negative impact on our lives. Our best chance for positive outcomes is to be aware of what we do, how we do it, and our clear intentions.

Learning in Focus

Learning is wound implicitly through the seven principles. Movement and learning are entwined as inextricably as the two strands of DNA in a double helix.

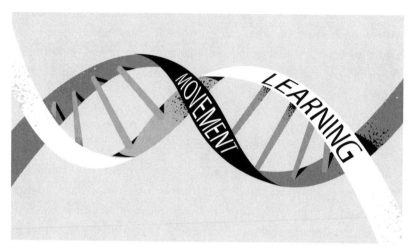

FIGURE 1: A model of movement and learning

Learning is a process that leads to change—the mechanism of adapting. In the space of one century we have moved from thinking of learning as the province of mammals to understanding that single-cell organisms, plants, and even machinery can be said to learn. We now know our nervous systems are massive ongoing learning networks, but they can learn many things that hinder rather than help, and it is only with the aid of attention and awareness that we can unravel the differences.

Most human learning takes place under the spotlight of **attention**—that moment when we bring our sensors (internal and/or external) to focus on a point of interest. Unlike learning, attention is hierarchical: the greater the stimulus, the more attention it receives. At its simplest, attention is noticing. When cultivated, attention is the beginning point of any investigation into the world inside and outside ourselves. It takes significant learning for us to shift attention deliberately, to block, expand, or focus attention. One mark of a maturing system is the ability to control attention in this way.

Awareness is the state in which we can expand attention to include greater amounts of internal and external information and make choices. For example, in an aware state we can be conscious of the chaotic noises outside the window, notice a rising feeling of irritation, and choose to let the irritation build or expand attention further to notice what thoughts are fueling the irritation. Awareness helps us expand knowledge of ourselves, our reactions, their meaning and consequences.[1] It is possible to live a conscious life with only very rare sparks of awareness. It is not possible to achieve our greatest potential without awareness because it is at the heart of self-creation. Awareness evolves after a long apprenticeship in controlling attention.

[1] Daniel Siegel, an esteemed pioneer in the field of mental health, refers to awareness as the "scalpel" that resculpts neural pathways, in his seminal work *Mindsight* (p. 133).

Using This Book
Baby Steps

We can learn a great deal from babies, if we duplicate how they learn with curious engagement in twitches and wiggles, endless repetitions, mistakes, delight, and frustration. Babies don't have strong muscles, so they must learn through ease, not force. They gradually transition as fluidly from lying down through rolling to sitting as they can move from curiosity through frustration and into pleasure. They have no words or ideas that separate their movements, no external concepts of "correct" or "ideal" or "should." They just have a stream of sensations that arise internally or externally and impel action. They must learn through acting and sensing their external and internal world, because there is no other option.

As adults we have valuable layers of cognition that a baby does not. We can direct our attention, our actions, and our reactions intentionally. We can label, categorize, and analyze after we have experienced. We can communicate all these things and share collective ideas. Yet these same cognitive qualities can also lead to predictions and associations that limit our ability to learn new things—they can lead to the limitations of the six blind men.

Once acquired we cannot leave cognition behind, nor would we want to. However, we can encourage ourselves and others to re-enter the more active sensate learning state of the baby, to great advantage. To relieve ourselves of the constant need to be right, look good, and have certainty is to regain some of that exploratory territory—rocket fuel for expanding our potential.

Words in Focus

The gap between words and meanings is an ever-present challenge for all of us.

Here is a very simple movement instruction: raise your arms above your head. If a group of people are standing inside a room, they will all raise their arms upward alongside their heads, so their hands point toward the ceiling. No problem here. We all appear to share the meaning of those simple words. But something different happens when people who are lying on the ground are asked to raise their arms above their heads. Some people raise their arms toward the ceiling, so their hands are now in front of them, while others take their arms alongside their heads, so they lie on the floor with their hands pointing in the same direction as the top of their heads. Such a simple word as "above" is understood differently depending on whether people orient the instruction to their body or to the environment. The action has made the divergence of meaning and orientation visible.

Some of the most useful information about people is hidden in the simplest uses of language and the simple actions we take. The more accurately we can listen, observe, and act, the more potential we can unlock.

Establishing a shared meaning is important. Some common words require precision and some uncommon words need explanation. From time to time, we will explain language pertinent to specific fields of knowledge, offering brief, pragmatic explanations sufficient for a non-specialist to grasp the concept. Some words and phrases are mere iceberg tips of enormous and maybe contentious fields of study, so we will clarify how we are using them. We hope that skirting the submerged mass will assist rather than insult.

You have already read a few of these explanations and clarifications: we draw your attention to them by highlighting the words themselves in the text. This enables readers to skim over explanations they do not need and to revisit those that intrigue or illuminate.

Practice in Focus

Embedded in this book is the hope you don't take our words as either gospel or garbage—you "Try It Yourself" (TIY). Each principle contains multiple suggestions for active exploration. The challenge of all learning is to understand concepts in many different applications and orientations, so the cul-de-sacs of situational learning don't form. Taking information from concept through experiencing to utilizing in multiple applications is the objective we hope to trigger by the TIY sections. But, for many reasons, you may wish to scan through first, before breaking concentration to try it. Or you may wish to skip the explorations and come back to them when you are in a better time and place to act.

As you continue through these chapters, you will notice recurring themes. The elements we touch on for one principle will occur and recur in many different perspectives. None of the principles happens in isolation, nor does one trump another in importance. They are not even separate from each other, except as a conceptual convenience. Each time you revisit the chapters the TIYs will change with the new dimensions you bring to them. This has been our experience and we hope it will be yours too.

It is our intention, in setting out this material, that people from many fields could find something of interest and value here. We have intended to explain enough to illuminate, but not so much to bog you down. We have aimed to explain abstract ideas in such concrete terms that you are tempted to actively explore them in your own ways.

The seven principles were first articulated for a Feldenkrais audience, but they are not unique to the Feldenkrais Method (see p. 172 for more about this method). They are the opposite of unique: we are describing patterns found everywhere throughout nature and woven into many practices. They are so obvious we are often blind to them. Understood consciously and practiced with awareness, they can have profound benefits for education, therapy, management, and performance applications. At their most basic, these principles are about our human potential.

Potential is not an unchanging absolute we are all born with. Our potential changes as we do. When the seventh blind man slid from the back of the elephant, his world view had changed, and with it all the limitations and possibilities of his life had also shifted.

BALANCE IS DYNAMIC

All movement requires a dynamic balance between stability and instability

A LONG SLACK WIRE suspended between two high posts, a quiet space, and a lithe young man—all set up to defy expectations of what is humanly possible. Li Wei leaps and cartwheels repeatedly across the slack wire.[1] Stunning, but it's just a warm-up. While still on the wire he is handed a strangely curved stick on which he balances, obliquely cantilevered to the wire. Finally, he is given a unicycle upon which he inverts himself into a shoulder stand and breathtakingly begins to pedal forward with his hands until he, the bike, and the wire create one continually adjusting image of moment-by-moment stability within an extraordinarily unstable system.

There may be only a handful of people in the world with the discipline and desire to reach Li Wei's level of skill. Yet most of us have experienced a small part of this feat. Somewhere in our personal history we

---

[1] There are several videos available on the internet of Li Wei's slack wire performances. His routine was included in the show *OVO* by the international phenomenon Cirque du Soleil.

have learned to adjust our balance continuously to ride something—a bicycle, a skateboard, or a parent's shoulders. We have at least the inkling of finding stability within instability—that is, dynamic balance. Of course we also do this every day. Each time we successfully take a step, we are finding a new point of stability over one leg, which attaches at the pelvis with a ball joint—a joint designed to allow continuous adjustment. And above that leg and pelvis is a chain of vertebrae, each with degrees of freedom available, topped off with a large ball (head) weighing more per square centimeter than any other limb in the body. Each step creates a wave of rebalancing through the hard and soft structures of our bodies.

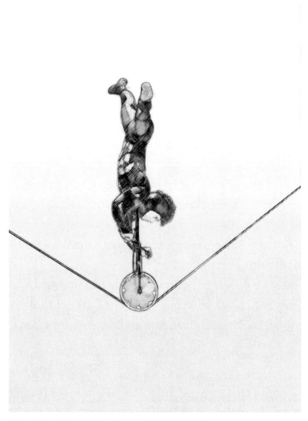

FIGURE 2: Li Wei balancing on the slack wire

The Beginning of Balance

Humans are the only mammals to have adopted this unstable upright stance as our preferred configuration. Babies must begin, from their day of birth, to learn the coordination that will eventually allow them to stand and walk. The first stage of this balancing act starts with the head.

Watch nurses or parents scoop a newborn into their arms. One hand must carefully support the baby's head, because humans are born without even the skill to do this. Through interminable trial and error, we learn to lift, balance, and orient our own head as a foundation for independence. The long muscles of the back extend the spine to bring the head up, while flexion muscles counteract to allow tilting, turning, and responding.

Flexing and extending are going to come up continually in this conversation, and they have very specific definitions in anatomy.

To **flex** is to bring two or more parts of the body closer, or to decrease the angles of joints. The muscles that create this action are called the flexors. For example, the biceps move the forearm and the upper arm toward each other and are therefore flexors. Abdominal muscles bring the chest and the pelvis closer, so they also are classed as flexors.

To **extend** is to take two or more parts of the body further apart, or to increase the angles of joints. The extensor muscles move in the opposite direction to the flexors. Rather than curling the body inward on itself, the extensors take us outward into widened, longer, flatter shapes. For example, triceps move the forearm and upper arm away from each other by opening a wide angle at the elbow joint, creating a long, straight arm. The large, long muscles down our back are extensors because they uncurl the torso, opening and lengthening the front of the body.

Put simply, a tightly balled fist is an example of flexion, and a flat, open hand is an extension. Every permutation between fist and flat is created by coordination between flexors and extensors.

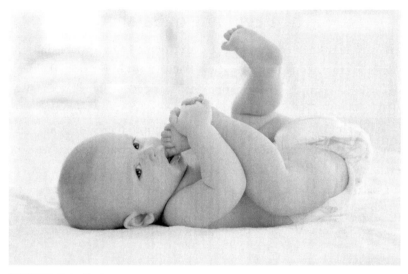

FIGURE 3: Baby flexing

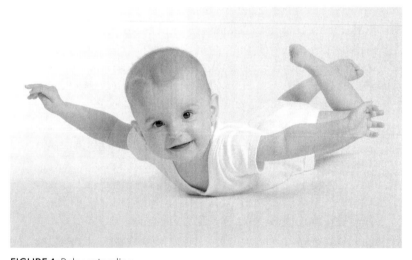

FIGURE 4: Baby extending

Babies practice coordinating the flexion and extension muscle groups in many orientations: lying on the back, on the front, and on each side. Complexity increases as babies begin to roll, to prop themselves on elbows, then knees, and then progress into crawling. Each stage requires finer coordination of the muscle groups, keeping that heavy head balanced freely on top of the spine so infants can face the source of their desire. Eventually, they learn to raise their head to the highest point over standing legs and take their first toddling steps.[2]

Flexing First

When we're lying flat, flexors curl us into ever-decreasing contact with the ground. As the shape and position of contact changes we become less stable but have more freedom to move easily in many directions. Babies must learn to use their flexors through the full range of lengthening and shortening to separate from surfaces and begin their rocking then rolling pathway to standing.

Little Rosa is a toddler, moving well through her milestones, but she needed help to get here. Rosa was born prematurely. She was well cared for by a vigilant medical team and loving parents. All was seeming to go well, until Rosa's inertia became apparent. First her mother noticed that Rosa seemed "flatter" than other babies when laid on her back. Rosa was neither waving her hands about nor watching them. She was reflexively stretching her legs but not folding them into herself. To fold we need flexion—the ability to curl—so elbows and knees come close to our centers. Rosa spread like a starfish and seemed unable to move from there. She needed to find her "abdominal crunch." To help her find it, whenever Mom or Dad changed her diaper, washed, or played with her, they helped her make simple flexion movements, such as curling her pelvis toward her chest—at slightly different angles each time—or playfully bringing elbows to knees or hands to feet, using touch and rhythm and sound to focus her attention. Her parents worked gently and playfully with her at every opportunity until eventually Rosa could draw herself into a comforting little ball and begin to roll, like all the other babies in the playgroup.

Rosa needed some extra help to kick-start flexion, but for most, this is unnecessary.

---

[2] Lois Bly has produced a marvelously comprehensive photographic and text description of the development stages in the first twelve months: *Motor Skill Acquisition in the First Year.*

Try It Yourself 1-1:
Revisit sucking and swallowing

Take a straw and a glass of water and begin to gently explore the relationship between sucking, swallowing, and breathing, then sucking, swallowing, and abdominal activity. The more gentle your activity, the more attention you will be able to spread to the bones and muscles, such as ribs and diaphragm. Use your hand on your lower belly to check for small muscle activations.

To deepen the action, choose increasingly dense or viscous fluids to suck through the straw. Keep the action soft and gentle, so you can experience more of the muscular activity needed for the more challenging action.

Now take your thumb to your mouth and begin to suck it. When is the sucking action most powerful—when you curl over so the elbows come toward the knees or when you extend your back, arching slightly to look upward? What about swallowing? If it is difficult to distinguish, play with the magnitude of the curling and arching, staying in each long enough to notice differences in how you suck or swallow, paying attention to the effort in your neck and lower jaw. More power with less effort is the equation you are looking for. It is the direction a baby will follow.

Imagine how many times, and in how many positions, you practiced sucking as a baby—and how you became stronger and more efficient at it.

In time, and as you were fed in different positions, you learned to use more coordinated movements of the whole body. The organization of abdominal activity, breathing, and swallowing became sophisticated enough to carry on these activities in many positions, diverse combinations, and with varying intensity.

Feeding and Coordinating

When a baby suckles at its mother's breast, flexing has begun. As the tongue and breath reflexively coordinate to draw in milk, other flexors of its tiny body are activated in small and instinctual movements.

You might be surprised that the beginning of dynamic balance lies in sucking. As adults we tend to take a very linear approach to learning new skills or improving established abilities. But that is not the path of implicit learning. "Life is what happens to you while you're busy making other plans" is a line made famous by John Lennon.[3] The same could be said of learning. While a baby is intent on nuzzling and feeding, it is also learning about orientation and coordination.

If babies have no neurological damage, and environments are safe and nurturing, they will usually acquire the necessary foundational skills without intervention. As babies respond to instincts, needs, and curiosity their learning expands exponentially. They discover their hands and feet. Their heads begin to turn and orient to different stimuli, gradually taking them into rolling so more of the world opens to their curiosity. As exhausted parents know, once an infant's coordination coalesces into crawling it is ready to explore everything and anything.

Moving Across the Ground

Finding balance on all fours is significant. The position provides enough contact with the ground to be stable, and enough elevation off the ground to be mobile. It is a template for action replicated with great success throughout the animal kingdom. The same four-point pattern for balance and motion underlies the movement of a seal, a mountain goat, and a mole—even though habitat, diet, and threats differ widely.

To start moving across the ground, animals must have a mechanism for creating both stability and instability. Too stable and we are stuck. Too unstable and we lose control: action becomes precarious. Every type of movement—physical, mental, emotional—needs a dynamic interplay

---

[3] This line was used by John Lennon in "Beautiful Boy (Darling Boy)" on the 1980 album *Double Fantasy*.

between stability and instability. It is important to understand this experientially, because in many instances we do the opposite. We brace, or rigidify, when we need to allow greater movement, and vice versa.

Meet Estelle. Over a period of twenty years, Estelle had gradually lost her sight, until she had only a vague awareness of light and dark. As the world disappeared, she found she needed guidance, but when she took hold of a guiding arm her whole body stiffened with fear of the unseen. She gripped with an almost clawed hand; she drew her arm firmly in to her side, and the muscles surrounding her rib cage contracted, as if ready to hunker down. This stiffening robbed her of responsiveness, making guiding difficult. The defensiveness she embodied physically also colored her social interactions, and she had gradually become reclusive. An old friend, remembering Estelle's past interests, cajoled her into joining a theatre group. As she was re-introduced to diverse movement and improvisation, her defenses altered noticeably. Her arms softened and even her vocal tone changed. She can now be guided easily and rapidly to where she wants to go, without the heaviness of her previous walk. Muscles that were once held tight to stabilize are now free to respond. The threats to Estelle's safety haven't changed, but her ability to deal with them has.

Try It Yourself 1-2: Sense how you stand and walk

Stand "normally" and notice what normal is for you. How far apart are your feet? Where does your gaze automatically rest— at the horizon, angled down to the ground, or above the horizon?

Easily lift one foot from the ground (not high) then put it back down. Repeat this several times, slowly enough for your attention to spread to the following queries: How do you transfer weight off the lifting foot onto the weight-bearing foot? Does your torso stay squarely to the front, or do parts turn? Is your gaze shifted left or right, up or down, by simply lifting your foot?

Many people will not adjust through their torso at all, so the whole body leans over one leg, like a tilting Eiffel Tower. Try it. You will notice your gaze moves dramatically with your head. Walk forward like this and your head will travel in a wide arc with each new step. Imagine what would happen if you walked this way on a narrow beam or tightrope.

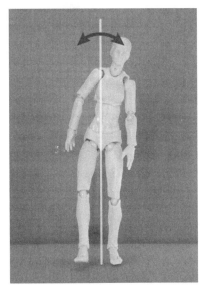

FIGURE 5: Tilting over one leg—head travels in a long arc

Gradually decrease the exaggeration of the tilt as you keep walking. You will find you can almost keep your head in the center, the shoulders square to the front, and move forward this way. Many people walk this way habitually.

Now stand still and lift your foot again. This time, as you lift, allow a slight turn in your torso, so the opposite arm swings slightly in front and toward the center line of the body, bringing the shoulder forward too. Can you notice your foot is now lighter to lift than when tilting like a tower? Go backward and forward comparing the two methods, until you can notice a difference in weight.

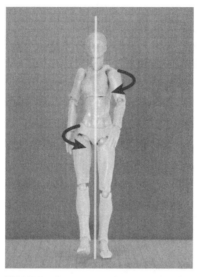

FIGURE 6: Stepping with rotation in the torso—head stays central

Begin to walk forward with lightly swinging arms and turning shoulders. Do you sense your opposite hip and shoulder coming forward at the same time? Notice how easy it is for your head to stay in the middle, so your gaze is steady. Would it be easier to stay on a beam if you moved this way? Reduce any exaggeration until the walk feels normal.

Now, as you continue this walk, begin to clench one fist, and allow the whole arm to brace in response. Keep walking and notice this effort rapidly spreading to your neck. If you hone your attention you may begin to feel tightening in the throat. Just stiffening one arm will change the mobility of your chest and the quality of your breathing. You may notice it influences the position of your head. Once again, switch back and forth between walking without and then with a stiffened arm; allow your attention to spread and detect the multiple changes.

Stand still again for a few moments. Revisit where you naturally place your feet now, and where your gaze falls. Has anything changed in your ability to notice?

Estelle's creeping blindness caused a chain reaction of limiting adaptations she was not aware of. The same is true for all of us. Events, environments, and habits change us during months and years, causing asymmetries that spread beyond the physical. The light and effortless movements of our early years may become impeded and overwritten.

Sensing Yourself

We need many ways to call our attention back to what we are doing: to question whether our habits are helping or hindering us. Balance is so automated in our bodies that we rarely notice, even when we have a problem. Tripping or misjudging a step height may perturb us momentarily but is quickly forgotten. The constant information stream coming into our sensory system and going out to our motor system is largely out of our consciousness. Yet we all have the means to improve the quality of this information. It is as simple—and as difficult—as refining attention to our receptors. Important cues for this are built in to the TIY you have just experienced, and in all the following chapters.

There are five groups of sensory receptors with key roles in balance. Playing with attentional shifts between the sensors offers a rich source of information to understand how we move now, and how we might start to move differently.

Teleceptors are in eyes, ears, and noses. These receptors feed in information about the external world, letting us see and hear *where* we are in space.

The **vestibular** system has receptors in the inner ear, giving vital information on the tilt or angle of our head in space and how it is moving.

Both teleceptors and the vestibular system depend on the freedom of the head for fine calibrations of balance. Giving attention to where your gaze lands helps provide information on habitual tilting of the head that might distort information. Noticing how lightly the head can glide for scanning, or whether the jaw is clenched, is an example of checking if your head is free.

Exteroceptors are in the skin and all organs that bring information from outside the body. When you stand and notice the contact between your feet and the ground, you are using exteroceptors. They can give us information about such things as pressure, contact, and changes as weight transfers.

Interoceptors are the interior sensory receptors. As you notice differences in breathing, you are using these.

Proprioceptors tell us about the position of our limbs in space and the amount of tension in our muscles.

Shifting and Balancing

Every step we take, every action we make, shifts our weight and challenges our balance. Any discipline that works with shifting and balancing load must have a concept of center of gravity and base of support—whether the discipline is launching a rocket to the moon, ensuring a roof stays on a house, or facing an opponent in a martial art.

The **center of gravity** is the point in any three-dimensional object where the weight (mass) above, below, and to the sides of the point is equal. Theoretically, if you placed an external support directly at the center of gravity, the whole object could balance on that point. Stationary objects have a fairly clear center of gravity, but a human body, which changes shape as we move, has a continually shifting center of gravity. As shapes become less symmetrical it is possible for the center of gravity to be outside the object or body—this is how cantilever construction works in architecture. When the center of gravity is external, it requires either significant bracing in the design or continual motion.

The **base of support** is wherever the object or mass connects to the ground (or supporting surface). Animals change their base of support continuously as the center of gravity shifts. If you have had the pleasure of watching giraffes drink at a watering hole, you will have seen these two concepts in action. As a giraffe lowers its great head and neck to the water, its center of gravity is moving down and significantly forward. The center of gravity is no longer over the standing base of support, so the giraffe must spread its front legs very wide and shift more weight into its back legs to prevent a survival-threatening nosedive.

So, what do these concepts mean in practice for us? First, the larger the base of support and the lower the center of gravity, the more power we must use to move. Think for a moment of the sumo wrestler: He squats close to the ground, with his legs set wide. He has a low center of gravity and a wide base of support. He is the epitome of stability and immovability—which is the crux of sumo. To lift one leg, he must transfer weight by leaning extensively to one side. The weight-bearing leg straightens as his head travels in a wide arc and the other leg becomes light and free to lift.

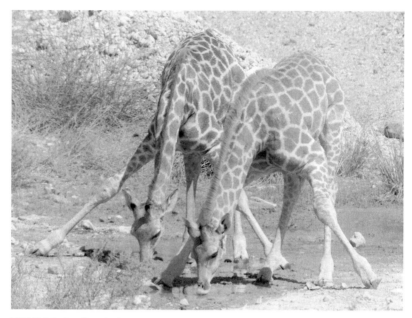

FIGURE 7: Giraffes drinking

At the other end of the spectrum is the ballerina *en pointe*—the smallest base of support a person could have while still on two feet (or one). With arms extended above her head, the ballerina takes her center of gravity to its highest point over this small base. She needs power and continual motion to stay in this extreme position because the merest tilt of her head can shift her from her center of gravity.

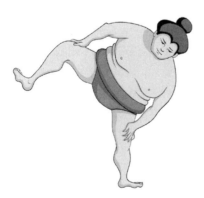

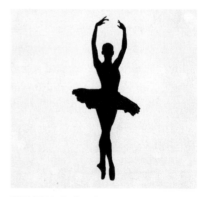

FIGURE 8: Sumo wrestler lifting leg   **FIGURE 9:** Ballet dancer *en pointe*

Both the sumo wrestler and the ballerina come from the elite end of human performance, where the art forms require an implicit experience of the principle. We have described moments of their practices, like snapshots, where the concept is hopefully clear and present. It's more challenging to illustrate absence. Yet to help people with difficulties, this is exactly what's needed—to recognize what happens when an organizing principle is either not present or not physically understood. As we mentioned in the first chapter, the therapeutic value is immense and will often be where the ideas are most usefully applied.

Fear of Falling

Follow in your mind Edward, an elderly man who is moving slowly and stiffly, using a walking frame. His feet are slightly wider than his body width and he leans forward a little with straightened arms to grasp the frame handles. All are indicators that Edward is looking for more stability. But remember the sumo wrestler and the giraffe: this gentleman has already achieved an incredibly stable position. His problem is not stability, but the effort required to move while maintaining this posture.

Zoom in a little closer. Fear of falling is associated with overactive flexors. We use flexion to calm babies when they are alarmed or upset. We place or swaddle them in a flexed position. Eventually they flex themselves to self-soothe. It becomes a refuge and response to anxiety for children and adults. The flexors bring the chin toward the chest. The abdominal muscles draw the ribs and the pelvis closer together, so we curl forward. To hold ourselves upright while the torso is curling forward, we must use significant effort in the extensor muscles of the lower back. To raise the head enough to look forward we must contract the muscles behind the neck. Essentially, we become locked in a battle between the muscle groups.

If you try that pattern yourself, in standing or sitting, you will quickly find there is little ability to bend to the side or twist—in fact the torso becomes quite rigid. To walk with this configuration feels effortful. Edward must lean sideways to lighten one leg enough to step it forward, an alarming teetering movement. Now his step becomes short and low to regain the ground and stability urgently. So every step takes great effort, creeps him forward minimally, and reinforces his anxiety about falling, exhausting him in the process.

Difficulties occur for so many reasons—disease, injury, trauma, or the insidiously slow impact of our habits over time. It can be very tempting for a person in pain, and the person who wants to help them, to get trapped in the circuit of naming and measuring dysfunction. But we are after something more pragmatic here, more accessible to every human who can observe, think, and feel.

Edward need not be an elderly gentleman; he could be a young man who has experienced a spinal injury, or a young boy with cerebral palsy. The same stability-vs.-instability pattern can occur in each of these instances. To move more efficiently and safely, each Edward must learn to be less stable or rigid through his center—his senses are telling him to brace, but he needs to move very particular parts of himself more. Just like Li Wei on his slack wire at the beginning of this chapter, each part of him needs to be ready to shift slightly to adapt to the demands of his environment.

Try It Yourself 1-3: Find mobility through the torso

Imagine a straight line on the ground. Just practice walking the straight line a few times, looking ahead but with your feet very narrow and close to the line. Now place your feet wider than usual and keep walking—noticing how that changes the feeling of your walk. You may be tempted to keep looking down at the line to stay straight, but that is not the aim of the game—you want to experience what walking a line, narrow or wide, with your head in its "normal" position is like; it is not important if you go somewhat crooked.

Now stand facing a wall and place your hands on it at around shoulder height. Stand with your feet more than hip-width apart and your knees soft (neither bent nor locked back).

How many ways can you find to change the curves of your torso?

You could try side-bending, so the right armpit and right pelvic crest come toward each other. Do you naturally include your head in this movement? Keep your face turned to the wall but allow your head to move in an arc to the right as you shorten your right side. See what happens to the spinal curve to accomplish this? The ribs along the right side must come closer together and correspondingly the left side must fan wider, like an accordion, or a C curve. How do you need to redistribute your weight over your feet and hands to make this easier?

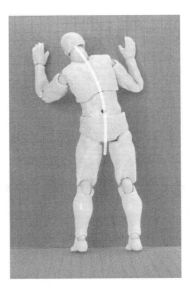

FIGURE 10: C curve—right armpit and right pelvic crest move toward each other

Try curving to the other side.

The more slowly and gently you take this exploration, the more parts—muscles and bones—you will be able to experience. Perceiving movement from the inside is not a skill most of us are trained in—it is acquired slowly. The brain must sort for sensations we have not included in our ideas of movement before. Keep the movements slow, even pleasurable, to allow your attention time to catch up and notice more.

The aim is to bring your attention to more parts involved in changing the curves of your torso—or spine. Can you create long sweeping curves from pelvis to head on each side, as well as forward and backward?

Is it possible for you to change the curve of your chest in one direction without changing your lower back and vice versa? What about taking the upper and lower spine in slightly opposing curves (an S curve)? Keep it small and soft to let your perception do its work.

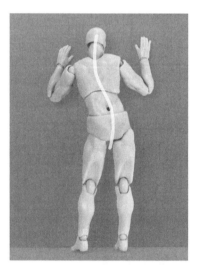

FIGURE 11: S curve—upper and lower spine in opposing curves

As you familiarize yourself with the possible changes in your spine, you can begin to spread your attention further. Can you notice as you curve in different directions how the weight shifts on your four points of support? One hand might become light with one arc, but as your curves change a different point lightens . . .

As you sense more, and begin to play with the size and range of movement, you may find it more comfortable to change the positions of your supporting hands and feet.

Can you sense how these different movements of your torso can move your head to different places in space, allowing you to face the world in many ways—up/down, left/right, and combinations of these?

Go back to walking along your line and see if your sense of stability has changed, or the ease of holding your head upright and central as you walk.

Every movement made with attention gives your information-hungry nervous system more data. Edward's system needs to know, in a very fundamental way, that it can shift through the center to create a safer, more efficient step forward.

It is important to understand that his walk will not improve by walking: that was not the way we learned as babies, and it is not the way we learn as adults. Instead Edward could explore rolling in bed, gradually discovering how to move his torso more and more easily. This is a wonderful safe arena for increasing mobility. To widen his experience of shifting weight and transitioning—important elements of walking—he can use sitting, then moving from sitting to standing. Both stable and unstable positions are grist for his system. His walk will improve by reawakening a sense of security and aesthetic pleasure in movement, in a system that had retracted into unconscious defensiveness.

We speak of balance as an ideal. We seek work–life balance, resolve to eat a balanced diet, and admire emotionally balanced people. Yet in all these instances, balance is not static. Balance is actively responding to constantly changing internal and external demands. Like the artist on the slack wire, we must keep moving, making small and large adjustments in the continuing process of balancing.

SKELETAL ALIGNMENT LIBERATES MOVEMENT

When the skeleton is aligned for support, large muscles are freed for action and movement becomes light and powerful

MEET THE TWO GRACES. They are in their mid-20s—both smart young women, but their lives couldn't be more different.

Grace A is Australian. She is an ultra-smart student, a shy but delightful young woman. She has spent many hours in front of a computer studying, watching videos, and playing games. She runs and cycles because she knows she should keep fit. But at an age of peak vitality Grace A rarely stands at her full, erect height. She can do so only for short bursts when she is paying attention. She has become progressively more shortsighted as the years go by and has consistently contracting abdominal muscles, tension headaches, and digestion problems. From side-on, it is obvious that Grace A's head is usually well forward of her central line, drawing her neck forward also. Her shoulders are rounded and pitch forward while the center of her chest caves and sinks backward to counterbalance the significant forward-thrusting weight—and this continuous countering goes on down to her locked (hyperextended) knees and fixed ankles. The force of gravity bearing down on her head and shoulders is not being effectively transmitted through an aligned skeleton. Grace A sags under the weight of gravity; her skeleton providing insufficient support, she seeks it externally by leaning on nearby objects or slumping into a soft, encompassing chair.

Grace A wanted a break after university and before taking up work as a teacher. She decided to go volunteering in Madagascar, where she met Grace M, a young woman of the same age, also a teacher. Grace M lives in a village where the wealthiest in the community have homes made of bricks. Bricks in her village are handmade from the damp clay of drained rice paddies and transported on the heads of women across the fields to building sites to be baked in kilns on the side of the road. Since they were young girls these women have been carrying loads on their heads, across muddy, rocky, or dusty fields, ditches, and hills. As young women they will carry all sorts of loads—buckets of water, piles of wood, stacks of bricks—often with a baby strapped to their back. To stay upright and moving under these increasing weights, the girls and women must effectively transmit the downward forces through their bones to the ground, as the large muscles stay free to move them over the challenging surfaces. Grace M may be a teacher, but she too carries heavy goods as needed in the different seasons. In fact, the first time the two Graces met, Grace M had been carrying a stack of sixteen wet, unbaked bricks on her head, out of the paddy fields, up the uneven footpaths, to the roadside kiln.

Grace M is a cheerful young woman, a little shy with strangers. She has very clear vision and stands, walks, and runs at her full height effortlessly and without thought. She moves fluidly and lightly across the rough landscape and can stand or squat unsupported for long periods of time.

Each Grace has adapted to a very particular environment. Neither of them has consciously chosen the factors that are shaping their very bones, but the sharp contrast creates a striking reminder. We are sculpted by our environment, our pursuits, and our attitudes to life. Grace A has many more life choices available to her than Grace M, but she does not realize how her choices are shaping her physically, nor the repercussions this shaping has.

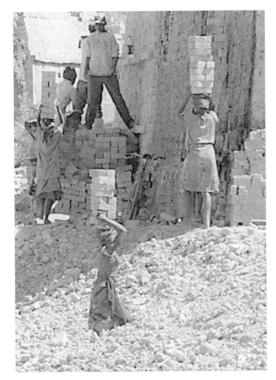

FIGURE 12: Madagascan women carrying bricks to kiln

Alignment and Action

The form we recognize immediately as human is created by our skeleton, a set of oddly shaped, articulated bones joined with connective tissue. It is theoretically possible to be so well aligned in certain upright postures that, if all muscle activity ceased, the skeleton would remain in place. This may only be theoretical, but it is a valuable thought exercise about efficient use of self.[1] There are practical ways to examine how close we are to this ideal, which we will touch on in this principle.

---

[1] "Use of self" and "self-use" are two common terms used in Alexander Technique and the Feldenkrais Method. Frederick Alexander was probably the first person to coin the phrases, referring to the way a person habitually coordinates themselves for actions. His seminal work *The Use of the Self*, first published in 1932, talks about use and misuse of the musculoskeletal system, with a focus on speech and performance.

The large muscles of the body are the headliners most of us recognize by their abbreviated names—abs, quads, lats, glutes, and so on. They are designed for moving our frames in space: dancing, swinging an axe, throwing a ball. These large muscles cross many joints and therefore cause several bones to move at once. For example, the abdominal muscles can cause the spine, ribs, and pelvis to move simultaneously. These muscles connect whole regions, so we call them **global muscles**. They are not well adapted for holding us erect for extended periods.

The small muscles, lying close to the skeleton, are the specialists in supporting the configurations of our skeleton. These stabilizing muscles cross one joint only, effectively "tying" one bone to the next, like the small spinal muscles attaching single vertebral joints. The actions of these muscles are local in nature; therefore, we refer to **local muscles**.

Yet another appellation for global and local muscles is "phasic" and "tonic," based on percentages of fast- and slow-twitch muscle fibers. The global, phasic muscle fibers switch on and off rapidly in powerful bursts, or "fast twitches." Local, tonic muscles can work for very long periods without fatiguing, because they have a majority of slow-twitch fibers. All muscles have a mixture of fiber types within them—fast for action and slow for endurance—but the proportions differ widely, creating muscles capable of both types of action but significantly more suited for one. Phasic-dominant muscles are more suited for action, and tonic muscles are more suited for support.

In summary, we have muscles that are best adapted to move us through space—described as global, phasic, fast twitch, or large—and muscles that are best used to maintain a stable configuration—described as local, tonic, slow twitch, or small.

For instance, if we rely on well-aligned bones and small muscles of our skeletal system to support and position ourselves, then our large, powerful muscles are predominately engaged in short-burst activity.

If, however, a person finishes their day with a stiff neck, sore shoulders, or aching back, they are most likely relying on protracted engagement of the large muscles to hold themselves upright.

Defying Gravity

If a body is well aligned in gravity, the local muscles switch on and support the structure, leaving global muscles to engage in large shape-changing actions. However, when not well aligned over the base of support, global muscles must become the support system for the structure. This is so fundamental it will be revisited in a number of organizing principles, in particular OP7 on pressure.

Gravity creates the need for bones, and muscles are needed to move the bones. Tellingly, our nervous system is not that interested in our bones. We can't sense the bones in the same way we sense our skin is cold, or a muscle is working. However, the nervous system is extremely interested in where the bones are in relation to each other, and in relation to surrounding tissue. We have many proprioceptors at our joints to feed back information on pressure and placement. We have interoceptors in flesh and organs around the bones. Anyone who has broken a bone knows it is painful, but the bone itself is not sending the pain message; it is changes in the tissues around the bone that excite the sensors of the nervous system.

Just as our skeletons are invisible to conscious sensing, so too is gravity. It is one of those fundamental elements of our environment that is so ever-present we don't notice it. We don't feel gravity, but the effects of gravity are written in every part of our bodies and impact all substrates of our thinking. What would upward or downward, heavy or light, even mean without gravity? Our physiology and psyche are so superbly gravity-adapted from birth that we require significant time and learning to understand the central place of gravity in our lives—how we use it, ignore it, or defy it.

For a moment, return to Li Wei's world of super-feats, where acrobats tumble through the air to land two, three, or more high on each other's shoulders. Would you classify this as a feat of strength, looking in awe at the strong man at the base of this human tower? Or as an example of dynamic balance, thinking of the acrobats landing on the shoulders of another? Or maybe both? Would it ever occur to you that the unsung hero in this event is the ability for bones to align on top of bones—the ability for weight from the top to transfer directly through bones to the ground even though the actual ground might be three bodies away from the acrobat? When weight transfers directly through the bone, what we experience is a sense of weightlessness.

Try It Yourself 2-1:
Align your hand, wrist, and forearm

Stand your elbow on a desk or table with the forearm pointing directly upward, the wrist straight so that the hand forms a direct line with the forearm, and the fingers curled over to make a light fist. Check that your forearm is truly vertical to the horizontal surface and not tilting forward. For the sake of clarity, we will say this is your standing arm.

Now place your other hand on the top of the fist and push down lightly so you can feel the elbow resting on the ground. The downward press can be gentle and at the same time move the standing arm so minimally you can feel the changing shape of contact between your elbow and the supporting surface. If your standing arm and hand are well aligned, you will not experience your wrist at all. The force will travel directly through the myriad bones at the joint as if the entire complexity of the wrist were a solid structure. If you continue this same movement in a gentle and inquiring manner you will find a "sweet spot" where the muscles of the upper arm, shoulder, and upper back are able to relax somewhat, because they have received a message that they are not needed in this activity.

While still pressing down lightly, bend the wrist of the standing arm a little in any direction and you will begin to experience the wrist. When forces change, our attention is pulled back from the junction with the ground to the joint that is no longer aligned. Keep the exploration light, changing the angle of the fist minimally, and notice the muscles of the upper arm and shoulder must reactivate because the force is no longer passing directly and harmlessly through the joint to the ground. We are keeping the pressure very light in this experiment, but imagine for a moment stress through the wrist, creating the need for extensive muscular bracing throughout the arm and torso to keep your wrist safe.

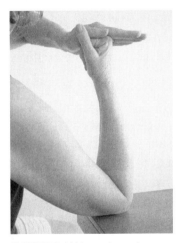 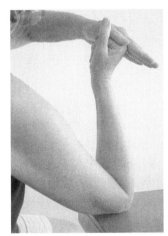

FIGURE 13: Wrist and arm in alignment to transmit force

FIGURE 14: Wrist at risk if force is applied through it

This configuration of the hand on top of the forearm is a good representation of skeletal support. When force travels directly through a straight line made by the hand and arm, you do not notice the parts: the fingers, hand, wrist, and forearm. You don't need great muscular strength to hold the structure in place. If the bones are truly well aligned, you can support significant weight on the fist and feel no stress. But should the alignment shift, that same significant weight will cause shearing stresses. You begin to sense effort as global muscles are activated to brace, because the local muscles are no longer enough to keep the form upright. If you continued to habitually do this with poor alignment, you would find pain generated in the wrist, forearm, elbow, and potentially the shoulder and neck.

Now extrapolate this out to the extraordinary daily feats of balancing a forward-weighted head on the top of the spine; adapting to the constant action of arms suspended from the necessarily unstable shoulder girdle; counterbalancing the delicately arranged forward-thrusting ribs that hinge with our spine. You are glimpsing the gravity-defying acts of stabilization undertaken by your musculoskeletal system, under the direction of your nervous system, each moment of your day.

It would be easy to think this discussion is about upright posture, but that is not where we are going. We are aiming at something far more interesting—access to power and the sensation of weightlessness.

For most of us, the word **posture** suggests a very static thing. If you listen to the echoes of your history, what do you hear when someone says "posture"? Chin up, chest out, bottom in, stand tall? Straighten up? Or maybe you visualize someone seated stiffly upright at a piano, a computer, or a dining table? Posture comes from the same roots as "post"—which is solid and immoveable—or pose—a fixed position.

We are most likely to strive for "good posture" when we feel we are being watched and wish to be seen at our best. The stress to impress might bring us toward our image of ideal posture, but it also tends to leave us stiff, wooden, and unable to think or speak fluently. We turn into very good posts indeed.

In fact, good posture is not a stand-alone concept. Think back to the giraffes (OP1): the posture that is essential for drinking is quite different from the posture for standing around. Similarly, good posture for modeling is very different from good posture for soccer, or good posture for glass blowing. They are really two different things: posture and acture. Artists' models need good posture when they pose. What a catwalk model, a soccer player, a glassblower, and everyday people need is good **acture**—efficient, well-aligned skeletal structure in action. But rather than using a word that is not listed in most popular dictionaries, we will continue the common usage of "posture" to cover both, with the caveat that we are always referring to a dynamic organization of the body in space, and not to a straightlaced set of imperatives pedaled by self-appointed deportment police.

Power and Alignment

Return for a moment to the idea of the previous TIY—the aligned fist, wrist, and forearm standing on the table. Mentally, or physically, lift the arrangement from the table, stand up, and arrange yourself as a boxer would. If you have managed to find alignment in the TIY, you have the perfect forearm arrangement for a powerful punch. In fact, boxers strap their hands and wrists rigidly into this alignment because small deviations risk injury and dissipate power.

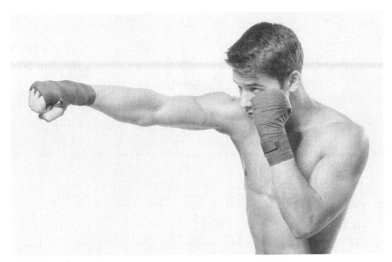

FIGURE 15: Boxer's wrist strapped to transmit force safely

If you wish to untangle the two concepts of strength and power, boxing is a great example. When you watch boxing, it is quickly evident that muscle bulk is not the deciding factor of the contest. Muscular strength is part of the training mix, but it is not the key to power (we will talk more directly about power in OP5 and 6). Boxers train for agility, endurance, and strength. They train to move fast and light—as Muhammad Ali described it: "float like a butterfly, sting like a bee." It's a beautiful description of experiencing weightlessness when weight transfers directly through our skeletal structure.

A traditional element of boxers' training is skipping rope. While it might look like just another way of training for endurance, it is much more than that. Skipping moves their frames directly up and down repeatedly and rapidly in the gravitational field, practicing effective alignment in gravity. The better aligned they are, the faster their feet can find and leave the ground with low effort, so the activity becomes more sustainable. The spiraling extensor muscles are long and passive as the feet connect with the ground, then shorten explosively to lift the body into the air like a rocket launch, where the extensor muscles switch off to start the cycle again.

The Maasai and Samburu warriors of Africa are famed for their ability to jump, in an action not unlike skipping rope with two feet together. Their ceremonial dancing is based on jumping, leaving the ground with a light and effortless spring like a gazelle. They appear to defy gravity as they bounce directly upward to heights most of us would view as impossible, and they can easily continue this dancing for hours.

Yet that same gravity that the warriors shrug off is a weight capable of gradually crushing our vertebrae into a breath-prohibiting forward stoop, if we are unable to transfer the force directly through our skeletons to the ground beneath us.

In our description of the two Graces we said: "we are sculpted by our environment, our pursuits, and our attitudes to life." Our skeletons are a solid, living record of how we have interacted with the weight of gravity throughout our lives. Just as weather, plants, and animals gradually change a landscape over decades or millennia, so environmental demands and personal activity change the architecture of our body over time. Falling out of a tree or colliding with a car may rapidly

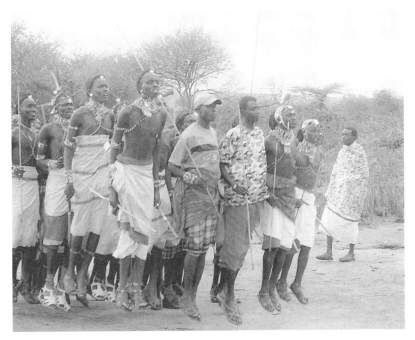

FIGURE 16: Samburu warriors dancing

change the shape of one or more bones. Less obviously, your choice of furnishings, pastimes, and professions make a difference to how your bones are shaped. Strong muscles constantly pulling at their anchorage sites cause bones to thicken and subtly reshape where the muscle attaches, just as poorly toned or unused muscles leave bone growth unstimulated. Strong, overactive muscles with inactive counterparts can displace bones from gravitational alignment, resulting in shearing stresses that cause cartilage and bone erosion.

With the advent of more imaging technologies, many people are finding out how unique their bony structure has become over the years. As a side note, though something within us may not look "normal," it is not necessarily the cause of pain. Pain and inability are more complicated than that.[2] Some people with extraordinary structural distortions

---

[2] *Explain Pain*, by David Butler and Lorimer Moseley, is a book of great wisdom with a twist of wry humor on the complexity of pain, its neurological origins, and pragmatic paths to recovery.

or damage from birth, disease, or injury achieve exemplary, active lives. Others may look like the templates for perfect posture yet experience pain constantly—and never feel capable of achieving their dreams.

An ideal structure has little to do with appearances. Historically when cultures have idealized appearances above function, painful and destructive practices have emerged to fit individuals into models of perfection. A functional ideal is tested in action, not images. So, an ideal such as "a structure capable of transmitting force directly without unintended dissipation" could be applied equally to a punch or achieving a life goal. If the kinetic energy supplied by standing tall with a high center of gravity can be used directly in running, digging, pirouetting, or creating what we want, then we can successfully live the life we desire. We will explore this further in OP4, when we discuss awareness of the absence of effort.

The Test of Transitions

Transitions are the best way to test the effective alignment of the musculoskeletal system. Transitions require both local and global muscles to be working effectively in order to transmit force directly through the skeleton without damage or loss of energy. Here is a way to understand how much energy you may be "losing" every time you stand up.

Try It Yourself 2-2:
Transfer weight from sitting to standing

Find a bathroom scale. The old analog-style scale is ideal for this, but most digitals will also do the trick.

Sit on a chair with the scale on the floor under your feet. Stand up and watch the scale as you do it. For most of us the indicator jumps well beyond our weight as we leave the chair. When we're completely standing, it will settle back at our weight.

An ideal use of the musculoskeletal system will show a different result. The weight over the scale will show a constant increase until you stand fully on the scale at your true weight without an overshoot. If you cannot do this, it will seem impossible. Some people will be inclined to believe this is just hyperbole. It is not. It is a way of moving yourself that can be learned.

The most likely people to achieve this initially will be those practiced in the martial arts, who understand how to move their center of gravity fluidly. But most of us, untrained in the attention this requires, have developed ways of moving that stick us in place until we build up enough effort to overpower the inertia and launch ourselves to standing. Apart from losing energy as mentioned, this is also a recipe for painful knees, eroding hips, and stiff necks.

Go back to the moment before you saw the indicator on the scale jump and practice this little transition several times. Can you notice your breathing? Is there a correlation between the labor of your breathing and the weight jump? Explore variations of bringing your weight over your feet. For instance, come forward while turning as if you were going to stand up facing one side; try the same to the other side. You could bring your arms forward in a long sweeping arc as if you were going to complete a forward dive, always watching how smoothly you can transition your weight according to the scale. Or bring your weight forward while gently and continuously swiveling your head.

When you have tried many variations with attention, return to the first way you stood up and see if it feels easier and lighter. Notice if anything has changed on the scale or in your breath. As you move away from the chair and the scale, pay some attention to any differences in your walk. It is not unusual to feel a shift in the weight and effort of your movement, even if you cannot quite label it.

There are many ways to improve the movement in this TIY, but for the moment it is an illustrative test for yourself. Some dedicated autodidacts may be able to learn this manner of moving with little assistance, but most of us do not learn alone very effectively; we do better with live instruction and an expert eye. Nonetheless, in the absence of either, if you can give up the ambition to achieve rapidly or perfectly, you may experience a new way to align yourself in gravity.

OP3

PROGRESS IS CYCLICAL

Evolving to stand upright with a 360-degree view of the world is a sequential progression that is revisited with each major movement challenge

LUCY PLAYS "ANIMAL SPOTTING" as a party game. As she watches people, she names an animal they resemble in movement and attitude. She has an uncanny knack for revealing interesting patterns through her observations. Like a young woman—skittish as a doe—tentatively scanning the canapés, ready to spring away from loud noises or unexpected movements. Another woman we call Lucy, discovered in 1974 but born about 3.2 million years earlier, highlighted our evolutionary lineage. Both Lucys point to something very fundamental about us, as individuals and as a species: each of us carries a record of the evolutionary stages within. We don't just carry it, we live it from the moment of conception. We begin as single-cell creatures, and during gestation we transition from invertebrate to vertebrate, through fluid-dwelling, and on to our births as air-breathing, land-based mammals.[3]

---

[3] Nineteenth-century biologist Ernst Haeckel coined a pithy little phrase summarizing this: "ontology recapitulates phylogeny." While Haeckel's theories became discredited in their literal form, the phrase remains useful figuratively in investigating development paths and has been used this way in a number of disciplines.

This chapter outlines the unfolding developmental path humans follow from wriggling to crawling to walking, through the developmental patterns of spinal, homologous, homolateral, and contralateral movement.[4] Each stage adds new ways to transfer weight and move through space. Each stage takes in more information from our environment and gives us additional ways to respond. In this chapter we play lightly with an evolutionary concept, but the underlying story is of humans attaining full height, with the ability to scan 360 degrees on all planes.

Spinal movements are very small responses to the pressure of the ground or the surface on which we lie. These are the movements of our invertebrate and early vertebrate ancestors: twitchings, wigglings, and wormlike beginnings of coordinated movement.

Homologous comes from the ancient Greek "to agree." In terms of movement, it means that the movement of the top half of the body "agrees with" or is roughly the same as the movement of the bottom half. Like reflections, the halves move toward and then away from each other. Frogs hop with this pattern.

Homolateral means "same-sided," so all the flexion happens down one side of the body, while the other side extends. As with homologous, the head moves with the curving spine, as a simple extension. Reptiles use this same-sided movement, also known as "ipsilateral."

Contralateral occurs when the upper right side now coordinates with the lower left side (and vice versa)—or opposing sides agree. So the right shoulder moves forward as the left hip moves forward. This diagonal relationship creates a twist or spiral through the torso. Now the head becomes free to move independently of the spine's direction. All mammals have at least rudimentary contralateral movement.

---

[4] It can be difficult to know who coined these terms, which are now commonly used across a broad range of movement disciplines, but a very likely source is Irmgard Bartenieff (1900–1981) in her *Bartenieff Fundamentals.*

Because writing is linear, development can appear to happen in a linear pattern, but it doesn't. All the stages are iterative. We may return to them at any moment of our development, for security, comfort, or a functional advantage. Individuals learn at their own rate, and in their own unique ways, stimulated or hindered by many variables. Some phases of development are drawn out, while others may appear to be skipped completely. However, used wisely, this map of the developmental sequence can give us insights into strengths, weaknesses, and options. It can also be a great resource for creative play and therapeutic assistance.

Deep in the womb, each person starts as a single-cell being. Around nine months from this singular beginning, a little human emerges from fluid surroundings into the dry-land and gravity-defined environment it will inhabit for life. And in this entirely new environment it begins to acquire the skills that will make it independent.

Spinal Movement

Our first movements in the external world are spinal. They happen during wakefulness and sleep and serve to awaken the spine, linking the first flutters of voluntary control through center to extremities. Many of us still use these expanding and contracting movements at the beginning of each day as we emerge from sleep into wakefulness: stretching, rolling, and undulating in the moments before we sit on the edge of the bed and launch ourselves into the day.

Spinal movements can be recognized in some interesting places, like getting in and out of tight garments, or extracting yourself from awkward spaces such as sleeping bags. These tiny spinal adjustments lie deep and somewhat dormant in many adults, but they have a very important place in maintaining healthy and adaptable behavior. Their proper use is a crucial element of good posture/acture, since they use the deep, local musculature to spread load and disperse the demands of movement across the whole spine.

Awakening your awareness of spinal movements offers many benefits. These minute movements, often hidden, enable you to balance with greater ease whether you are active or at rest. Hip-hop dancers learn to pass these undulating movements up and down their torsos and across limbs—to the delight of their audiences. Spinal adjustments form the solid core from which to make all other movements.

Try It Yourself 3-1:
Explore spinal movements

Take a towel and roll it up lengthwise. Have it lying parallel beside you on the floor. Now wriggle yourself on to the rolled towel without using your elbows, heels, or head as leverage points to get there. That is, you don't push into any of those outer points to raise any central part of you. Can you do all your maneuvering with your back—lifting, rolling, and sidewinding—leaving your limbs and head free to simply slide? In this way, bring yourself to lying lengthwise on the rolled towel.

Your head and spine should now be in line, and your arms flat on the floor at your side providing you with balance. The rolled towel should provide a gentle feedback ridge along the length of your spine. If it creates discomfort, then decrease the height by unrolling the towel a little. Bend and raise your knees so your feet are standing (semi-supine position).

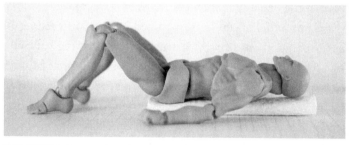

FIGURE 17: Lying semi-supine on towel

Lightly, sequentially press parts of your spine into the towel. Each vertebra has small degrees of movement available, so an undulation of gentle pressing can gradually be passed up and then down the spine. Likewise you can lift small sections, passing a ripple of lifting up and down the spine. Take time to explore both lifting and pressing. It is unlikely you will feel specific vertebra, but you will be able to feel sections of the spine pressing or lifting. Pause periodically and simply imagine what the movement might feel like. With time the sections will become smaller and more precise. Your movements can become subtle, so the breath is undisturbed.

Pause. Take a moment of rest to notice your comfort level in this position now. Has the sensation of lying on the towel changed at all?

Lifting and pressing into the roll are small awakenings of spinal extension and flexion. The spine can also move sideways. Please use the same subtle investigation to find the small side-bending movements that can similarly ripple up and down.

(Achieving these light undulations can take time. Return with curiosity at different times of day, or different parts of the week, until you feel the aesthetic pleasure of discovering a primal movement that began before birth.)

When you are ready, ease yourself off the towel. Take your time to notice if more of your torso can wriggle and move onto the flat floor. For some people, the floor may not even feel flat anymore. You may be aware of lying more completely on the floor, and the floor itself may feel mysteriously softer.

Find your way to standing. Scan your spine for some echo of the small differences you found on the roll. Notice if there is any quality difference to how you stand and move—even if it is a subtle difference you cannot label.

> Remember that both the pauses to notice and the reflection moments are very important, and most easily overlooked. Noticing difference is the absolute foundation of learning. Difference is data for our nervous system, the information that stimulates new connections and strengthens old. Attention to differences of quality, efficiency, and satisfaction separates learning from exercise.

Homologous Movement

When the small pressing and lifting spinal movements can be produced with some consistency, they grow larger and more coordinated, connecting larger sections of the body in one movement. At this point, homologous movement can appear. It's created when the top and bottom halves of the body can curl toward each other. On our back, the hands can now take hold of the knees or feet. And when we roll onto elbows and knees, things can get exciting. The upper and lower limbs come together in a flexing action and then release like a spring as the extensors activate. At first this is an inchworm-like motion, but as a baby learns to coordinate this with power, the homologous pattern becomes more like a frog or bunny hop.

This pattern is a baby's means of propulsion. The head rocks forward and down, bringing sufficient weight over shoulders and arms for the pelvis and legs to become light enough to slide forward, then settling the weight into the pelvis and legs so the head and shoulders can lift and move forward. Babies begin on belly with elbows and knees and gradually elevate to hands and knees.

Like all the developmental patterns, it remains in our repertoire all our lives. Spotting where and when you, or others, use homologous movement can be a very helpful game. The big hint is that the head always stays in the center. It neither tilts sideways toward a shoulder nor rotates. In homologous movement, the head's only trajectory is forward or backward.

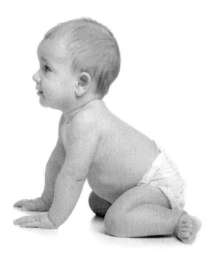

FIGURE 18: Baby sitting with the homologous pattern

The homologous pattern feels very safe and secure for movement—so safe that we use this when at our most fragile, for instance when disease or injury has damaged our ability and confidence to walk. Using a walking frame takes us back to this very early top/bottom pattern. The frame takes the weight of both arms, allowing enough lightness in the legs to move each foot forward. Once the feet are directly underneath, in a solid stance, the weight is transferred off the arms into the feet, so the frame can be lifted very slightly and moved (or wheeled) forward.

In elite sports, this very early movement is used for rapid access to power. It gives us large forceful bursts, like the launching movement of the downhill skier or a swimmer off the starting block, the mighty downswing of the champion axeman, or the upward thrusting lifts of the Olympic weightlifter.

Try It Yourself 3-2: Revisit a homologous crawl

This is best done on a floor with a smooth shiny surface. Friction is not your friend in this TIY, so find a place where you can slide.

Lie on your stomach with your elbows drawn in and standing underneath your shoulders (like a sphinx). Can you put enough weight into your elbows to draw both your knees up underneath you? You will find that to do this, it is easiest to drop your head downward, so the top of your head comes close to the ground, and you could maybe look beneath your torso toward your legs.

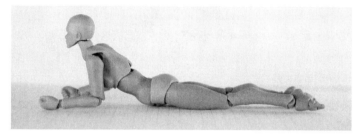

FIGURE 19: Lying like a sphinx

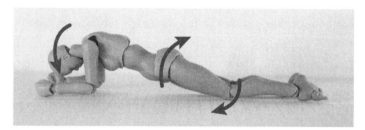

FIGURE 20: Weight on elbows, drawing both knees forward as head drops and pelvis rises

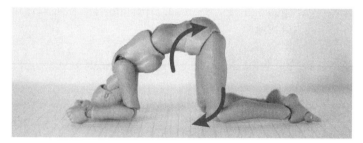

FIGURE 21: Crawling position, weight forward

If you have been able to draw your knees under you, your pelvis will most likely be high in the air. You will be almost standing on your knees, but the weight is still forward on your elbows. (If you couldn't quite coordinate that first movement, then please cheat and place yourself onto knees and elbows. You will eventually be able to do this from the lying position.) Now begin to lower your pelvis down toward your feet as if you were going to sit back on your heels. You will find this moves most of your weight backward and invites your head to lift and look forward. Your arms lighten and lengthen so you can either slide or move your elbows forward a little.

As you repeat this, you can move forward in hopping or sliding movements. First the elbows slide forward; then they steady and accept more of the body's weight as the knees lighten and can be drawn forward. The head and the pelvis have a seesaw relationship with each other. When the pelvis is high toward the ceiling, the head is low toward the floor, and vice versa.

When the head is toward the floor and the weight in the elbows, you can strongly flex the torso to draw the knees forward. When the pelvis moves back and downward toward the heels, the flexors should release fully, allowing the large extensors to raise the head, lighten the arms, and extend them forward. It is from this simple switching of the flexors and extensors that the power comes.

Some young children with a disability, for whom this is the only accessible crawling motion, can hurtle around a space with great alacrity using this homologous action. It is often accompanied by a wide smile and even a chortle, because humans find great joy in moving powerfully and of our own volition. It is delightful to witness children's discovery of self-propulsion: this first sense of the world as theirs for exploring.

An important feature of this configuration is the concentrated focus—all attention is converging on the subject directly in front of us. Think for a moment of a cat preparing to pounce. Its head is low and eyes unwaveringly on its prey, not dissimilar to a downhill skier waiting for the starter's signal. The cat crouches, weight on the forelegs, hind legs bunched, ready—but not yet irreversibly committed—for a fast and powerful launch.

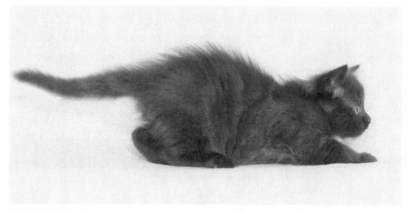

FIGURE 22: Ready to pounce

The homologous configuration focuses our attention tightly on what is immediately in front of or inside us, and can be our refuge in extreme concentration, preparation, fear, or anxiety.

Homolateral Movement

When something off to the side finally catches our attention and stirs our desire to reach for it, we are ready for homolateral movement—the awakening of right and left. Homolateral movement is marked by a baby being able to contract on one side while the opposite side becomes a long corresponding curve. In other words, we can draw the right elbow and knee together, while the left hip and shoulder move further apart from each other. As the baby explores this more, it will begin to shift its weight across to the longer side, allowing the shortened side freedom to lighten, lift, and finally reach out to the object of curiosity or desire.

The world on both sides now begins to be within reach of a baby's curiosity. There is another boon. As the reaching hand lands on the ground and finds stability, it now becomes a supporting arm onto which weight can be transferred, and a new way to move forward (or backward) has begun. This manner of progress, shifting weight from one side to the other, is a more efficient crawling pattern than the energy-hungry hopping of the homologous phase.

With advantage also comes disadvantage. The greater efficiency of homolateral movement comes at a cost to stability. Undulations (spinal) or rocking forward and backward (homologous) are very stable patterns. Now as the head moves further and further to one side, the torso must counterbalance by shifting substantially to the opposite side, creating challenges to balance along the way.

Reptiles are masters of the homolateral movement. To counteract the inherent instability, they remain close to the ground and have long tails that extend their base of support. Babies, however, are gradually decreasing their base of support. They must spend a long time, with many variations, learning to move homolaterally. On their backs, they playfully reach right hand to right foot, and left to left. They roll onto their stomachs and return to their backs by shortening one side then the other; they creep backward then forward and commando crawl on elbows and knees before progressing to the higher, less stable hands-and-knees position. All these variations are stimulated by the head shifting significantly to one side and then swinging to the other.

When this ancient pattern of movement becomes well learned and integrated into our system, it changes from a demand on our balance to a first refuge when balance is challenged. Sailors will use this one-sided movement as seas get rough and the deck of the ship begins to roll and tilt. Close to home you may see shoppers side-bending with the weight of a grocery bag and moving forward with homolateral gait to steady themselves. Fledgling acrobats will use these movements when first learning to move on a balance beam, tightrope, or slack wire.

Increased speed and agility are worthwhile benefits of the time spent in this movement phase. We have access to power, but with greater efficiency. In elite sports, you will find this type of movement used by the slalom skier, elegantly and swiftly shifting weight from one side of the body to the other as they move around the poles of their course—or in the serve of a good tennis player, flexing downward on the racket side, allowing the throwing side to be long and open in preparation for a large and rapid contraction as the pattern reverses.

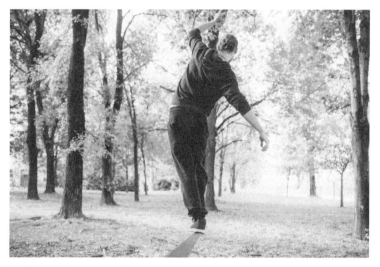

FIGURE 23: Homolateral movement on slack wire

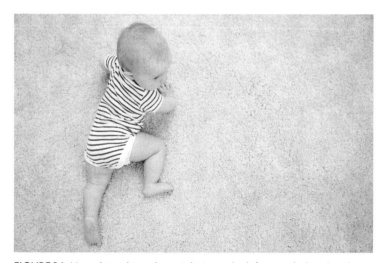

FIGURE 24: Homolateral crawl—weight is on the left, so right hand and knee can lift

Try It Yourself 3-3:
Revisit a homolateral crawl

Again take to the floor on elbows and knees.

Allow your attention to settle on something far to your right. If you take your head and eyes further and further to the right, you will notice your right shoulder comes closer to your right hip and your left elbow begins to lift from the floor. As this shortening of the right side happens, the ribs on the left side can expand, and the spine makes a large C curve, long and convex on the left and concavely curving on the right.

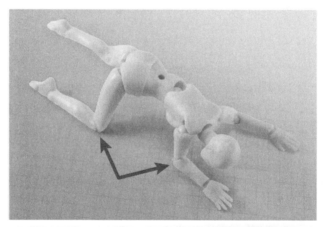

FIGURE 25: First stage homolateral crawl—looking right with weight on right

As you do this curving you will notice you could take more weight into the right elbow and knee, but that would not help you reach for the object of interest. It would eventually topple you. Babies go through this stage, repeatedly and with great frustration. Gradually they learn to shift their weight to the left while their head swings lightly to the right, so they won't fall.

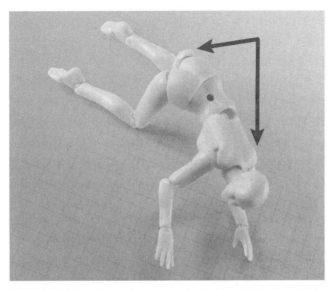

FIGURE 26: Mature homolateral crawl—looking right with weight on left

Continue curving to the right and then back to straight several times, noticing the weight shifting onto different points of your limbs. A moment comes when your weight can shift completely off your right side onto your left elbow and knee. At this point the right arm and leg become weightless enough to lift and move freely. You could reach the right arm out to the object of curiosity, or you could place the reaching arm forward on the ground ahead of you. If you find yourself with the right elbow placed ahead, your torso will have straightened and begun to lengthen on the right so you can shorten on the left. You can now scan leftward and begin the process again.

You can try this crawl on elbows and knees, hands and knees, hands and feet, and even in walking. Pay attention to various aspects such as where the weight shifts, which limbs are now heavy or light, which side is short or long, and what you can see or reach.

In everyday life we use this movement quite regularly without ever noticing. It is an important part of our repertoire.

Lauren is a bright, bubbly girl, full of curiosity, but born with brain damage that has limited her development and her independence. So many therapy sessions have come and gone in her young life, but one has always stood out. It was the day she learned to shift her seated weight from right to left: the day she was first able to transfer weight to her left buttock while shortening her right side by dipping the right shoulder and raising the right buttock slightly. For the first time in her life she could reach her right hand beneath the slightly raised right buttock, slide it under her right thigh and out again. If you have kinesthetically followed that movement as described, you may have guessed at its importance. With this new ability Lauren won herself an important piece of independence. Her caretakers could now take her to the toilet, close the door, and wait outside, because she could clean herself without assistance. If you have ever lost that ability in adulthood, for whatever reason, you will have had a glimpse of what that meant for her.

Contralateral Movement

During purely homologous and homolateral actions your head moves as a simple extension of the spine, like a tail. The central focus that was a distinct feature of homologous movement is disrupted by homolateral movement. The alternating side-bending motion of the spine sweeps the head from side to side and gives us the ability to scan. For the next level of sophistication, the head must move independently from the spine. This requires contralateral coordination.

Contralateral movement is the movement of mammals. While it still uses four points to stand, each limb is capable of separate and coordinated movement, and the head has become free to orient independently of spinal motion. Because it is so energy efficient, mammals can range over enormous territories, using the contralateral movements to walk, trot, lope, or jog for great distances.

Developmentally a human baby's nervous system has integrated a mass of information about forward, backward, up, down, and sideways motion. It has been building an intricate image of body parts and their relationships. First a baby's world was an undifferentiated whole in which it could simply twitch and wriggle. It then "discovers" upper half and lower half for homologous movement. Homolateral movement opens an entirely different range using our sides, but it is not until contralateral that we can use one side of the top half, with the opposite side of the lower half. Finally the infant can begin to move each limb independently, in a diagonal or spiral coordination. The left hand will move forward with the right knee, and the right hand can move forward with the left knee. This creates a gentle twisting movement as shoulders rotate in one direction while the pelvis rotates in the contrary direction around a central axis—the spine. At the top of this axis the head moves freely, largely independent of the movements of the spine and body beneath it.

At this point a baby can lie on its belly and raise its head, so its eyes can rest levelly on the horizon. It can roll fully to its back without taking its eyes off the horizon—a feat very few adults can do. In other words, it would now be capable of a full 360-degree scan of the horizon while rolling, crawling, or dropping itself into a seated position. From this point a baby can stand up, the most precarious and versatile position of humans.

At a full stand, we have our greatest potential energy. Movement becomes less of an effort because we are harnessing the full challenge of gravity to help us move in whichever direction we wish. The head can nod forward and backward, it can incline or translate sideward, and it can rotate vertically on its axis. Ultimately it can maintain a fixed point and smooth trajectory as the spine continuously changes its curves beneath it. We can sustain a focused point or wide

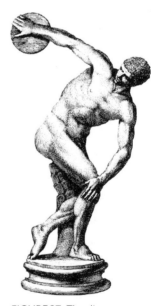

FIGURE 27: The discus thrower—a spiraling contralateral pattern

peripheral vision. During this whole progression, our central nervous system has kept learning, creating new pathways, adapting for greater complexity and finer control.

Examples of contralateral movement are found in every field of human endeavor. But for a frozen moment that captures the essence of the spiraling, contralateral pattern, it is hard to go past the ancient Greek statue of the discus thrower or *Discobolus*.

Try It Yourself 3-4:
Observe people walking

Rather than do a movement-based TIY this time, it is time to increase your powers of observation. Take yourself to your favorite people-watching place—bus stop, café, community park, shopping mall, or anywhere you can sit and observe many people walking by. Look at how people move. Whose head stays in the middle while their torso rotates (contralateral)? Whose head tilts side to side as they walk (homolateral), and whose head moves forward and backward, birdlike, as they step?

Watch people's backs as they pass. Can you notice whether they rotate their shoulders or their pelvis? Maybe you will see people who get shorter on one side or the other, or whose spines tilt forward and back with very little rotation. Notice some heads remain level while others move up and down, as if people were getting taller and shorter as they walk. What happens when people are carrying or pulling a weight with one of their arms?

As you watch, considering the simple patterns we have mentioned, you will begin to understand the extraordinary array of movement possibilities and habits. You are seeing the unconscious habitual patterns we all adopt as we grow and live. The four patterns of movement we have discussed are merely points along spectrums of potential; it is unlikely you will ever see one

> pure pattern. You will see a great range of mobility and immobility, asymmetrical limpings, hitchings, tiltings, and turnings. Try to remain free of judgment of good and bad, or assumptions about *why*.
>
> People move in all manner of ways, for all manner of reasons, and understanding that diversity is of huge value. Observing others can be enormously helpful for better observation of yourself. If you make special note of unusual movement and try it out when you are back home, you will have begun to unpack an endlessly fascinating study of individual diversity.

This TIY can be a launch pad into understanding how some people get exhausted easily, experience persistent pain in specific areas, or even injure themselves recurringly in the same place or on the same side. The combination of observing others and experimenting with self-use is fertile ground for both therapeutic application and development of your own potential.

Moving in Cycles

There are many ways of explaining or investigating the developmental sequence. We have chosen to look through an evolutionary prism, emphasizing the orientation of the head and adjustment to gravity. You could also understand this development sequence spatially, in terms of planes and axes of movement (more of this in OP5). This would invite an exploration of each phase as an expansion of movement into the three dimensions of space. It is a wonderful framework to use, which opens many different vistas for people who are fluent in the concepts of spatial relationships.

We have also mentioned the intellectual and emotional components of these patterns. As you observed people in the TIY, it is possible you noticed different emotional tones and levels of alertness in the passersby. Movement, thinking, and feeling are inextricably connected, with a complexity that is difficult to capture except, perhaps, obliquely. One approach to understanding these connections, not as generalizations but as possibilities, is through personal histories. The following is a personal recollection that was evoked by an exploration of the developmental sequence. It is also a rather neat summary of the whole.

William, now an astute young teacher, was once an undersized and timid boy. At age ten he went to a school adventure camp for the first time. He had a strong fear of heights and wasn't too keen on water. Both the things he dreaded appeared in one event on the first day at camp.

A challenge was laid out for the students that began with crossing a creek via a log. The log spanned the creek banks a meter above the water. Some of the kids walked along the log without any concern—heads held high, one foot placed in front of the other without hesitation, scanning the far bank for what was next before they were even off the log.

Some students needed more time. Their arms were flung wide to give themselves better balance, and their heads swung widely from one side to the other as they proceeded hesitantly. They tended to move forward in a staccato rhythm, one sliding step at a time. A few stopped partway across, dropped to their knees, and continued in a safe and steady crawl to the far side, where they could finally step off with a slightly sheepish smile of relief.

Then came William. This was a huge challenge for the small boy, and after only two steps William was onto his hands and knees. Even that proved too challenging, so finally William seated himself, legs dangling down on both sides, and both hands firmly on the log with extended arms. William crossed the log by pushing down into his hands and hopping his bottom forward, in a slow and effortful progress. His eyes down, he stayed focused on the next short distance he could achieve with each hop. Despite hearty encouragement from the teachers, when he was finally across, he rose from the log feeling ashamed and unwilling to look anyone in the eye.

For William the greatest surprise from this event came at the end of the day when the group gathered around the campfire. William was singled out for his bravery. His fear had been painfully obvious to all. That he had been smart enough to find a way to keep moving, despite his fear, had earned him the respect of the organizers. According to William's recollection, that day has significantly informed his approach to teaching, and perhaps even his choice to teach.

Whichever way we describe development, there are natural progressions. One level of achievement creates the base for the next, but no level is ever extinguished. Sometimes that first level is the best, most effective level to use, and that is what your nervous system will default to. While the use of terms such as "progressions" and "levels" might seem to imply a hierarchy, there is no hierarchical preference in our nervous systems. That is an intellectual conceit. The bias, in a healthy nervous system, is toward efficiency.

Each development takes us toward greater efficiency. We begin to use the challenge of gravity to our advantage. The further we raise ourselves away from the ground, and the greater the flexibility in the torso, the more we can use the potential energy created by a higher center of gravity. At full height, with our head and eyes able to scan 360 degrees of the horizon, we are able to spread movement through all parts of ourselves. That is, we are capable of myriad combinations, not just of body parts but of all components of movement, to cope with diverse situations both internally and externally.

This chapter has been about an unfolding pattern of development that doesn't require intellectual input. It requires a safe, nurturing, and stimulating environment. Ironically the development of our intellectual abilities can hinder our full and efficient use of these patterns in adulthood. Our wonderfully plastic nervous system has no filter for "best practice." So we learn—through imitation, socialization, and major or minor traumas—to behave in ways that impede our most effective movement and counteract some of our best early development. For this reason, we need ways to continually reassess our own movement, and reawaken the pleasurable pursuit of our full potential. We trust you will find some tools for this in the next chapter.

OP4

QUALITIES REFINE SELF-DIRECTION

Attention to quality of movement creates an internal reference system for exploring movement, recognizing unconscious habits, and learning new ways to move

DIANNE GREW UP IN a house with many mirrors. Not only were there mirrors on the walls but people who consistently reflected on her posture, appearance, and actions. She showed talent as a dancer and was encouraged to train. Again she had many mirrors and teachers for feedback and correction. Everything that Dianne consciously learned about movement was based on how she looked. Then came a choreographer who did not talk about shapes and lines but directed her to find feelings and sensations to portray to an audience. Dianne was lost. She had never developed her attention to the internal experience of movement—in fact she had consciously suppressed it, to reduce the unpleasant aspects of long hours in training. Experiencing her actions as sensations and breaking the reliance on mirrors took a long time. It was both uncomfortable and liberating. At first she was full of doubt, but she learned to listen to internal information with growing confidence. As her trust in her own senses grew, the uncertainty and fragility she had thought were normal diminished. Years later, Dianne now pinpoints this as a pivotal change in not only her dancing career but also her life.

Every human starts life learning through sensations. Sight, hearing, smell, touch, and taste are just a small selection of what humans can sense. We have interoceptors for temperature, pressure, spatial arrangement, balance, satiety, and more. Yet when we leave infancy and begin our long, formalized education we silence much of this direct sensory information. We prioritize thinking above sensing and accept theoretical truths above embodied experience.

External authority and feedback are important, but disproportionate reliance on them results in a life always mediated through another's perspective. Many people never learn to trust themselves.

The question that worried Dianne as she tentatively began to listen to herself was: "How do I know I am doing it right?" It's an excellent question. When we are exploring new territory we need markers for safety, confirming we are going where we think we are going, doing what we think we are doing.

Because trial and error is the foundation of all learning systems, we want our mistakes to be safe and fruitful. Four qualities that can guide us are: absence of effort, absence of resistance, presence of reversibility, and freedom of breath.

Seeking these qualities redevelops sensate learning: the same process that brought you from a babe in arms, through rolling and crawling, to a mischievous toddler—without instruction, demonstration, or a how-to manual.

To re-enter the childlike state of unconcerned exploration, adults must deconstruct some of their most practiced approaches to movement as exercise. Fast, habitual, or goal-oriented movements make it very difficult to pay attention to quality, to notice your own sensory world.

This chapter is about developing a quality of movement and attention that allows us to make valuable distinctions. Distinctions are the rich data a learning nervous system feasts on.

Absence of Effort

It will most likely seem an odd idea to define something by what is not there. Yet absence is an important learning concept. That which is very familiar goes unnoticed except in its absence. As the adage says: "You don't know what you've got until it's gone." Through absence we learn vital information that habit and familiarity have concealed.

> And what exactly do we mean by **effort**? Simply using greater force, or more exertion, than is required for the result produced.

Riya is a "gym junkie." She loves fitness classes and individual workouts, but she has been unsatisfied with her stamina. She decided to ask a trusted friend to observe her during a workout. Her friend noticed out that every time Riya lifted weights or did strength work, she began to breathe very audibly. She would grimace, pursing her lips, inflating her cheeks, and noisily push air out or pull it in. So her friend asked Riya why her breathing was so different with this type of exercise. Riya had never noticed, so she became curious. She discovered when she focused on strength, she clenched her jaw and tightened her throat. This made her feel she was working hard, but rather than giving her more power it was constricting her breath. These habits were so strong it took continuous attention to avoid them. Attention takes time. You must slow down and do less to notice more. That was not easy for someone dedicated to pushing herself; it felt like going backward. But the dividends came as Riya continued. Her neck and shoulders became less stiff, her movements became smoother, and her strength improved, without the familiar feeling of hard work. She easily surpassed the point where she had plateaued for so long. The missing stamina had been hidden beneath all the extra efforts she had been unaware of until her friend asked one little question.

When we cease effortful movement, our skeletal frame takes its full height and width, because the compression caused by co-contractions is released. When the skeleton is at its full dimension, and the muscles that move the bones are free to shorten and lengthen as required (OP2), then the load of any task can be spread throughout a responsive system. There is no mistaking the experience, because the limbs immediately feel lighter and the work easier. We are free to use the entire array of long bony levers, muscular springs, and other mechanical advantages of our form and frame.

As Riya discovered, effort can be ingrained to the point of invisibility. We are rewarded from an early age for making obvious efforts, for doing more than we can do easily. Effort is considered praiseworthy and is synonymous with both "trying hard" and "doing your best." Well into adulthood we will work with greater effort than is truly required, to impress real or imagined observers. Those things we learn early and reinforce often are very difficult to notice, even if they are causing harm and limiting our options.

Massive work can be done without experiencing effort. When every iota of force used by an athlete is directly converted into synchronous movement, they can appear to move with superhuman ease. However, when we are having difficulties, the use of force is not contained within the desired movement, so neighboring and even distant parts of our bodies become enlisted in effort.

Try It Yourself 4-1:
Sense how effort spreads

Clench one fist, tight and hard, and hold it, even increasing the level of effort as you hold. Notice how many other parts of your body also become tight or rigid in response. Most people will find that their jaw clenches; contractions occur in the throat that narrow the breath channel; ribs and chest become rigid.

Release the fist and notice what parts of your body also let go—whether obviously related or unrelated to the fist. If you go back and forth—contracting, holding, and then releasing—you will soon notice how infectious effort is.

If you now take a heavy hammer or saucepan and grip it tightly enough to swing it and bring it down rapidly (but safely), you will not experience the same rigidity that simply tightening the fist caused. When we have a functional outlet for the force, we do not rigidify our frame in the same way as we do in purposeless effort.

Effort narrows our field of attention. We fixate on the object of the effort to the exclusion of other information. Conversely as we decrease effort, our capacity to notice sensory feedback increases. You can see this demonstrated in the niche world of safe-cracking competitions. Champion safe-crackers are practiced in decreasing all forms of sensory distraction including physical effort. Fingers, hands, arms must all work lightly with agility and responsiveness. The body must be alert and balanced without effort, and all sensory distraction quieted, so the smallest tactile and auditory changes can be detected by the safe-cracker.

Try It Yourself 4-2:
See effort in the mirror

Sit in front of a mirror.

Close your eyes and think of something you find effortful. It could be doing sit-ups or getting suitcases off the top shelf or solving a calculus problem. Imagine yourself doing this effortful activity, then open your eyes and look at your face. Can you see the signs

of effort—tightening of the skin around the eyes and mouth, fur-
rowing of the forehead, and maybe clenching of the teeth and
jaws?

Now close your eyes and think of something that is easy and
pleasurable to do. Again really imagine yourself in the activity,
then open your eyes and see if you can detect the differences in
your face now. You may even have felt the differences as your
facial tonus changed between the two thought experiments,
before you opened your eyes.

Just thinking can create effort in us. Conversely, thinking twinned
with attention can be a means to decrease effort.

Riya continues her investigation of decreasing effort at the gym.
For most people this would be a strange place to practice effortless-
ness; however, it is a fabulous playground for experimenting with
spreading load, using less force to achieve better results. She can take
sneak peeks at how others work and compare how they coordinate
themselves to achieve an exercise with how she is doing it. Now that
Riya has noticed excessive force, she can see it everywhere.

Absence of Resistance

Both effort and resistance are about the use of force. Effort is felt
when we use more force than necessary. Resistance is experienced
when opposing forces meet. Resistance brings us to a full stop, much
like finding a boulder in your path. You could pit your strength against
the boulder for little or no reward. More effectively, you could find
another way around the boulder, so you could reach your destination
without exhaustion or damage.

Resistance appears in many forms and levels of our existence.
At the purely physical level there is obstruction, like the boulder, or
friction.

Try It Yourself 4-3:
Explore turning

Place a soft, fabric-covered chair next to a seat with a smooth, solid sitting surface, such as a wooden chair.

First sit on your wooden seat and turn to look at something behind you. As you repeat the same action several times, give yourself a chance to notice how much your head, neck, and spine are involved in turning. Can you feel that turning is easiest if you allow your pelvis to help? If one thigh slides forward on the seat, your pelvis can turn slightly; weight shifts onto your feet, which enables more rotation all the way up the spine, allowing your head and eyes to see farther behind.

Now sit in your comfy chair and turn as far as is easy. Can you sense the resistance to movement this environment creates? The resistance means less if you can be involved in the movement easily. On a soft, high-friction surface you must rearrange yourself significantly to slide a thigh forward, rotate the pelvis, and turn.

Athletes and their coaches constantly search for smarter ways to decrease wind, water, or ground resistance by adapting form, uniform, equipment, and so on. Yet we give little attention to resistance we meet consistently in our daily environments.

Soft lounging chairs are a delightful creation for relaxing after a big day, but they also represent how we unwittingly accept environments that limit us. Rather than consider the restriction of soft, enveloping car seats, we blame aging, or a stiff neck, for our difficulties in looking behind to change lanes or reverse.

We also experience resistance internally. At the positive end, it is protective: our muscles and nervous system detour us around breaks, sprains, and other physical impairments, virtually splinting the injury and neighboring areas to prevent us from causing further damage. We must find another way to move. Anyone who has woken from a bad night's sleep with a wry neck has experienced one of these blocks. Our temporarily immobilized head and neck force us to find alternatives for turning left or right. Thankfully wry neck is usually a short-lived experience. However not all resistance is so obvious, short-term, or protective.

Gavin is an amateur runner. He runs for pleasure but also to relieve the stress of a busy office-bound job. Increasingly he'd been having small, niggling injuries, and he noticed they were mainly on his left side. He also observed there was significantly different wear between his left and right shoes. Finally the injuries interfered too often with his ability to run and he sought some assistance. A very gentle investigation of how he shifted weight between his left and right leg showed he was unknowingly resisting the direct and full transference of weight to his right leg, as if he was protecting the right side somewhat.

This discovery unearthed a memory from his youth. As a boy Gavin had badly sprained his right ankle during a cross-country run. With the impatience of youth, he had ditched his crutches early and started training as soon as the swelling had subsided somewhat. Now, as an adult, it seemed his gait was still protecting his right foot from the impact of full weight-bearing. It was a subtle and long-practiced habit that was completely unconscious.

Young Gavin had used willpower to override the discomfort of his partially recovered ankle. Like effort, willpower is praised as a virtue and highly encouraged. Developing willpower is an important step in individuation and maturity. Yet there can be downsides. Because he was more motivated to be on a school team than to patiently give his body healing time, Gavin had unconsciously adapted the way he ran, and many years later he was still running that way, though all need to detour around an injury was long gone.

The issue of motivation is significant. Each of us deals with conflicting motivations—arguably the most fertile and invisible cause of resistance. A quick example is waking to an alarm clock. Many would prefer to roll over and go back to sleep, although they know they should jump up and start their day. As a result, they lie immobile for long minutes, neither sleeping nor leaping out of bed. We become snared between two actions when contradictory impulses arrive simultaneously at our skeletal muscles. If one impulse is stronger or clearer, we act; if not we are blocked. This phenomenon is not unique to humans.

Siva is a beautiful, sleek dog built for running and hunting. He has been very strictly trained. Occasionally Siva accompanies his master to the local café. When his master goes inside to order, Siva goes to the curb and sits on the very edge, looking at the tree-lined park across the road. Then something rather bizarre happens. Siva begins to spring, with both his front legs lifting and falling as if to leap, his head and chest straining forward, but his haunches remain firmly seated as if glued to the pavement. The conflicting motivations are clear in Siva's movement: the front half of his body is ready and actively doing everything required to dash across the road; his back half, however, is obeying his master's command to "stay."

Our outward manifestations may be subtler, but our conditioning can be as constraining as Siva's training. Opposing motivations are often so deeply imbedded in our socialization that they remain out of awareness. If we listen carefully, we hear examples in language. Words like "ought," "should," or "must" can be good indicators of conflict: they signpost a "but" lurking in our thoughts and feelings. Alternatively we may discover conflicting motivations by paying closer attention to sensory cues. Siva will never consciously examine which action he wants to fully commit to, but we can.

A little curious attention daily to the presence of resistance—environmental or internal—can reap large rewards in regaining or improving energy and ability. The next quality is ideal for sparking curiosity.

Presence of Reversibility

On the surface, reversibility is a very simple quality. It is the ability to stop and/or reverse a movement in any moment, without special adjustments. If we think only of physical actions, it seems a relatively straightforward concept. Once practiced, however, reversibility can provide rich veins of information about habits and patterns in all spheres of behavior.

A common action every mobile person does many times a day is moving from standing to sitting. If you watch carefully, you will notice that many people lower themselves to a certain point and then drop the remainder, especially if the chair or sofa is quite low. Falling or dropping are irreversible and jarring. Lowering reversibly is much kinder on joints, spine, and temperament.

Try It Yourself 4-4:
Sit down with reversibility

You can choose any chair for this, but the easiest would be a kitchen or dining chair.

Slowly begin to lower yourself as if to sit in the chair, and every few centimeters (or inches), stop and reverse with exactly the same trajectory, speed, and muscular tone you descended with.

The toughest part is a few centimeters off the seat. If you can smoothly lower your pelvis to lightly touch and then lift away again to stand, without a tiny grunt, or feeling increased work in your thighs or changes in your breathing, then you are achieving reversibility. If you noticed changes of speed, breathing, or effort then here's some further tweaking.

Transitions, like standing to sitting (and vice versa), are fundamentally about how we transfer weight. In this case the conundrum is how to keep weight centered over your feet while your pelvis moves backward toward a seat. Conversely it is how to smoothly bring weight forward when you transfer from a seat to your feet. An answer to this conundrum is counterbalance.

As you lower yourself to sit, lightly extend your arms forward and allow your head and chest to follow them. As your upper torso inclines forward, your pelvis gradually reaches back. (Many people keep their eyes fixed on the horizon, which tends to lock the head and spine rather than permitting the necessary incremental changes in shape.) Your arms will be farthest forward when your pelvis is touching the seat. At this point you could do a simple seesaw, gently tipping forward and back, noticing your pelvis raising off and lowering to the seat with an easy reversibility. When you have played with the seesaw a few times, allow yourself to sit back fully onto the seat, noticing how your weight shifts from your feet and into your upper thighs and pelvis.

Try a small variation next time you stand from a seated position. Begin your transition by inclining your head and chest so far forward that your knuckles can reach toward the ground in front of your feet. Keep your eyes on your hands as they continue to reach forward and upward in an arc, drawing your weight forward over your feet until your pelvis lightens and lifts. With the weight fully on your feet, your arms and eyes fluidly continue the arc upward until your upper torso and pelvis come to a centrally aligned position.

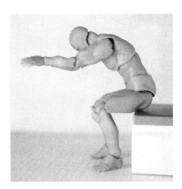 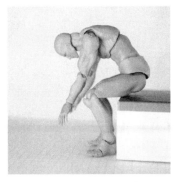

FIGURE 28: Transition to/from sitting—arms extended forward

FIGURE 29: Transition to/from sitting—arms extended downward

As you play with this transition you can gradually decrease the exaggeration of extending your arms. Parts of your spine will reawaken to their role in counterbalancing as you transfer weight up, down, back, and forward.

There are so many more variations we could suggest. These directions use the frontal plane, but you could explore how the sides of the torso can bend or turn through parts of the transition to make it lighter. For many people a slight spiraling motion is easiest, so you come to your feet ready to move off to either the right or the left. Increasing the ability to keep changing focus and orientation gives us many more options for practice.

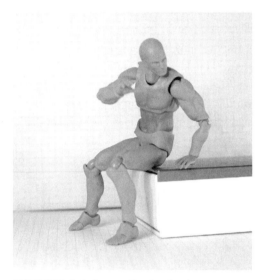

FIGURE 30: Spiraling motion to stand

When we are met with resistance internally or externally, we must find another direction/trajectory, and reversibility is a means for finding it.

Coming from sitting to standing slowly can be easy, light, and pleasurable. It is graceful. We sit and stand so many times each day that we have many opportunities to reinforce ease and lightness—or the opposite.

"Slow" has been mentioned several times here and it is a challenge for most of us who have grown up in societies that promote busy, driven role models. Slow is an important speed for attention: small parts of a movement made slowly and reversibly can provide masses of information.

Mei's job requires her to speak publicly. She travels the country presenting at conferences, seminars, and other public gatherings. She has always found large venues with large audiences quite easy; the sound systems are good, and the audience is distant and relatively anonymous. Small towns with little old halls are often entirely different. The audience members are fewer and closer, and their faces are visible. The amplification systems are not always reliable, leaving her with only the natural acoustics of the hall. Over the years, little venues had made her nervous, and if she presented in several consecutively, she would become hoarse. A couple of times Mei had lost her voice completely.

Despite the nerves, Mei loves her work, the travel, and the people she meets. So she took her loss of voice seriously. She began researching. One of the most important things she did was to take short comparison videos of herself presenting to an empty living room and then to a small, real audience. By chance there was a horizontal line at head height when she recorded herself in front of the live audience. She noticed that just before she began to speak, she somehow became shorter. When she was standing still, waiting to be introduced, her head was fractionally above the level of the line. The moment before she began her first sentence her head dropped beneath the horizontal line and stayed there. Mei couldn't quite believe what she was seeing. Her head wasn't tilted, her knees weren't bending; it was as if her whole torso somehow shortened.

So Mei began to experiment with this small part. She taped a grid to her wall so she could video herself against it, and she began to experiment with getting taller and shorter in the moments before she spoke. She found the best way to duplicate the shortening she had observed was to tighten the tummy muscles and the muscles at the back of her neck. It meant the plane of her face moved forward just a little toward a vertical grid line, and the top of her head dropped beneath the horizontal line. As she reversed this, she discovered she was releasing muscles not just at the back of her neck and in her abdomen, but even the muscles around her rib cage. In her research she had found a lot of discussion about lengthening this and contracting that, but seeing and feeling it was a very different experience. As she practiced going back and forth between tall and short, she began to feel and hear the difference vocally. When her face moved forward, her neck and throat tightened, and the sound became rougher.

Mei continued her self-experiments not just in private but live, in the moments before she began her presentation. A remarkable side effect emerged. As she became more skilled at noticing the extraneous contractions that led to hoarseness, she also noticed how much earlier the abdominal contractions happened with different audiences. Gradually Mei made a link between the anxiety she felt in front of small audiences and the increased work in her abdominal muscles.

When you are working with reversibility, the moments of delight are when you begin playing with the boundary. Finding the teetering line between control and going too far allows you to explore the distinction between the moments when you can still stop or change the action and the moment beyond which you cannot. It is at this boundary we can become really engaged, and the potential to learn about ourselves is laid open.

Freedom of Breath

The fourth quality involves the most ever-present and elusive quality of all—our breath and our breathing. Just as mercury expands and contracts with temperature, so too our breathing changes with physical, emotional, and mental fluctuations. Yet, unlike mercury, our breathing is not just a passive indicator but also an agent for adjustment.

As a gauge, breath is so sensitive you could use it alone to guide yourself to excellence, or freedom from pain and struggle. However, it is a rare person who, when asked to observe their own breathing, does not begin by changing it.

The variations in breathing are diverse—volume, rhythm, placement, speed, and multiple combinations of all. It occupies an important space between our unconscious and conscious control.

Holding your breath is perhaps the very first observable sign of discomfort, effort, perceived danger, or maybe an emotional shift

Try It Yourself 4-5: Breathe

Choose a physical exercise that is just slightly challenging for you—something like a push-up, sit-up, chin-up, or picking up a heavy object. Get yourself into a position to do the exercise, then notice what happens to your breath at the very beginning of the movement. Did you hold your breath, or need to change your breathing radically, to complete the action? Notice what it is like to attempt the exercise again without disturbing or holding your breath. Your habitual posture will relate to the halting of breath, so how do you need to change your configuration to keep breathing smoothly?

Now think of something you really don't want to do—some task that you "should" do but you find unpleasant. As you think of that task, noticing how you feel about it, what happens to your breath? If you could detect a change, then experiment with what it is like to think of the task yet keep your breath smooth and unchanged. Do you still feel the same way about the task when your breath stays calm?

When we discussed absence of effort, we spoke of Riya's discovery that she habitually constricted her breathing during weight training. Somewhere in her history she had equated the sensation of constricted breathing with heavy lifting. The entire pattern of how she worked with weights was involved, and as she unraveled the mystery of her audible breath, her strength and stamina improved. In other words, as she freed her breath she liberated potential.

As our posture changes so does our breathing; as our mood changes so does our breathing; and as our thoughts change so does our breathing. So every individual, social, or cultural rule about how we should look posturally, how we should act in particular environments, or what we feel compelled to achieve will have a repercussion in our breathing.

When we finally notice differences in breathing, the temptation is to apply rules for correction. There is no end of advice available for how and when we should breathe to achieve this or that. Athletes, singers, and asthmatics, to name a just a few groups, are bombarded with instructions and techniques for breathing. We are suggesting an alternative response—that you change what you are doing rather than how you are breathing. As we change the configuration and manner of what we do, the breathing will take care of itself. Unhindered by conscious intervention, a light, full breath is a quicker indicator of the right direction than any other measure.

As Riya continues to explore how better to lift weights, she might adjust her base of support whether she is standing, sitting, or lying (OP1), or investigate how her alignment adapts to the weight transitioning through space (OP2); she could experiment with the freedom of her head to scan 360 degrees (OP3), to name just a few arenas of attention that might help her lift with more ease. The first indicator of improved organization in any of these is increasing freedom of breath.

Freely moving breath is an exquisite cascade of events involving all our physiological systems as it carries air into and out of our bodies. A hand placed gently on any part of the torso should be able to feel the cycle of breath, without auditory or visual confirmation. No matter what the position or exertion level, the tide of breath can reach all parts of the torso (though not in equal magnitude) during well-organized movement.

While we are not advocating breathing exercises or techniques, if you have never considered what your natural breath—unhindered by accumulated psychological and physical habits—might feel like, then you may be excited to learn that breathing can be investigated with the same attitude of curiosity, attention, and awareness we are proposing for any aspect of movement.[1]

---

[1] In *The Breathing Book*, Brad Thompson lays out pathways to rediscovery of your natural breath in simple steps.

Exploring Qualities

By now you will have noticed that it is impossible to illustrate a single quality without also mentioning the others. A change in one will change all.

Attending to the four qualities can be applied to all aspects of movement, to minor details or major patterns. To familiarize yourself with them, however, it is best to start with activities you have no ambition for, approaching the challenges with playful inquiry, not striving for success. If you don't know where to begin, then challenging yourself to use your nondominant hand during a familiar task is a great place. For example:

Try It Yourself 4-6: Find clues in the non-habitual

Find a pair of scissors and a piece of paper. Make some cuts in the paper, paying attention to the sensation of cutting the paper. What are you aware of? Most of us focus on an outcome, like the shape of the line we are cutting, and notice little else. We rarely notice the action itself unless we are experiencing a problem.

Now put the scissors in your other hand and do the same thing. Leaving aside the fact the cuts look crooked or jagged, notice what the experience of cutting with this side feels like. So much more than the hand is activated as you cut. Your whole arm is involved, as is the way you hold your neck and head, and where you shift your weight. Many people tighten their jaw and thereby inhibit breath. If you attend closely enough you may even find your attitude (thinking and feeling) is different when you cut with this side.

As you go back and forth between the habitual and non-habitual hand, differences should become clearer. You could investigate all four qualities. When do you "try hard"— that is, feel effort or experience resistance? You may not be able to reverse by un-cutting paper, but can you easily stop and reverse the action of your hand, arm, shoulders? Can you pay attention to your breath through both left- and right-handed cutting? Does your breathing halt or become shallower during either?

You may surprise yourself with how swiftly improvement can take place with this exercise of attention to sensation. There are many opportunities to change handedness in daily chores and discover a wealth of information through similar investigations. Try cleaning your teeth or toweling yourself with the nondominant hand, and so on.

It has been mentioned before, but it is worth reiterating—every aspect of life is based on movement. So it is no great leap to understand that quality of life is directly connected to quality of movement. Yet day-to-day living tends to obscure this connection. Many of us learned early in life to pursue socially rewarded goals at the expense of our internal sensations. Searching for easy and pleasurable options was regarded as laziness. Recovering attention to sensory qualities can be tremendously useful in unraveling chronic issues that may have limited you for years, and it also offers an entry point to that enchanting and joyful state—flow.

HEAD GUIDES AND PELVIS DRIVES

Efficient movement requires a head that is free to orient us, connected by an adaptable spine to the power generated at the pelvis

GIANNI MIGRATED TO AUSTRALIA when he was a young man. This short, stocky man worked hard in a shop he built from nothing. Now, at the age of ninety-six, he spends much of his day sitting in a nook of the store on an upturned milk crate furnished with a small cushion. People come and go. He nods, smiles, converses, and occasionally dozes on his sturdy make-do seat. He keeps an eye on his store, but mostly enjoys the random interactions with family, staff, and customers as he wishes. When he wants to go somewhere, he leans forward, bringing his weight over his feet, stands up, and heads off down the road with slow precision, often forgetting the walking stick that his family would prefer him to take.

The cheetah, fastest of land animals, also rests watchfully most of the day. Choosing an earth mound to attain effortless height, it maintains vigilance with the least expenditure of energy possible—head erect, balanced sphinxlike over its forelimbs, hind legs lying long and inert on the ground. No bulging "six-packs," quadriceps, or buttocks give evidence of the explosive power available to this elegant animal. The resting breath, scanning eyes, and swiveling ears are the only signs of engagement in its body. Should opportunity for a successful hunt present itself, everything changes. The haunches mobilize, gathering then propelling the body forward in a powerful surge. Eyes fix on the prey, orienting head and body in rapid pursuit of a weaving, fleeing animal.

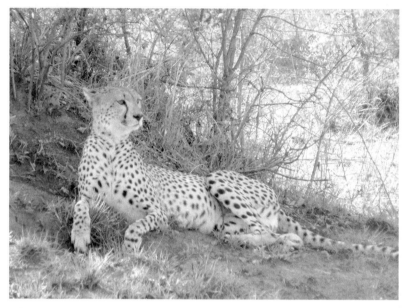

FIGURE 31: Cheetah resting watchfully

A ninety-six-year-old man and a cheetah—it's not where we would normally look for similarities, yet they are here. Both maintain a keen interest in their environment but by necessity are very frugal with energy. They spend most of their day in an attitude of restful alertness, head upright and scanning freely. When they have an urge to move, there is no struggle to rearrange themselves for standing: the pelvis becomes the locus propelling legs and torso through space in the direction set by the head.

For humans, and all land-based vertebrates, this special relationship between the head and the pelvis, mediated by the spine, provides the orientation and power to stand, to walk, and to do whatever else we choose in our three-dimensional world.

Your Guide: The Head

We spend the first two or more years of our lives learning to bring our heads to the highest position possible for our structures (OP3). At full height we have greatest access to information. Our teleceptors, the receivers of stimuli from a distance, are all located in paired organs on our heads—our eyes, ears, and nostrils. Our teleceptors receive information about what is "out there" and where we are in relation to it—that is, our position and location in space—our orientation— vital information for any action or response.

Full, upright height brings with it another special gift: maximum potential energy.

Energy, in physics, is the capacity to do work. A boulder balancing on the tip of a mountain has enormous **potential energy**. Should its balance be disrupted for any reason, its potential may be activated—converted to kinetic energy (the energy of motion)—if it falls with great speed and force down the mountain. A boulder lying on the valley floor has no potential energy.

Like the boulder on the valley floor, a head at rest on a pillow has no potential energy. However, a head at the pinnacle of the standing body needs very slight positional changes to activate potential. Additionally we have much more weight at the front of the head than at the back. This means the head, when upright, is always under gravitational pressure to move forward and down, counteracted by our spinal (local) muscles holding it up and back tonically. Every movement of the head requires adjustments throughout our musculoskeletal system to reinstate balance. Even the questing movement of the teleceptors subtly prepares the torso for action.

Of course if we bind our heads by global muscular contraction through the neck and shoulder region, we limit our easy progression from stillness to movement. It is analogous to cementing the boulder to the top of the mountain: you limit access to its potential energy, and a significant force would be required to liberate it.

With the head balanced at the peak of our standing height, we have easiest access to motion combined with orientation.

The primary motion of the head is rotation.

Try It Yourself 5-1:
Find the axes of rotation for your head

Place one finger of each hand on either side of your upper neck just behind the earlobes (there is a nice nook in the rear lower curve of the ear for this). If a rod (axis) now ran between those two fingers, your head could nod forward and backward around the imagined axis; your nose would draw a vertical arc running down toward your chest or up toward the ceiling.

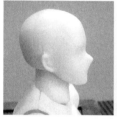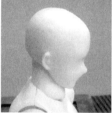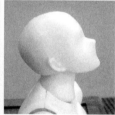

FIGURE 32: Head tilting front and back on horizontal (left to right) axis

---

Now, at the same level, move one finger round to the center at the back of your neck, just below the skull, and shift the other finger forward to the tip of the nose. Turning your head around this imaginary rod will tilt it left and right—chin swinging left as forehead swings right (and vice versa). Again, the axis is horizontal, but this time the action is lateral.

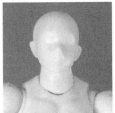
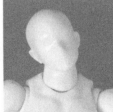
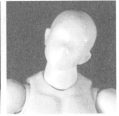

FIGURE 33: Head tilting left and right on horizontal (front to back) axis

Finally, take one finger to the top of your head and imagine it is creating a rod joined to the top of your spine. Now turn your head around this vertical axis, so your face turns left as the back of the head swings to the right—your nose would draw a horizontal arc left or right around the vertical axis.

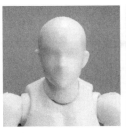
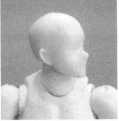

FIGURE 34: Head turning left or right around vertical axis

The next part is a "wee challenge," so approach it with a playful attitude and see how you go. Turn your head rightward around this last (vertical) axis until your face is looking to the right. Hold this position as you move your fingers to your earlobes and then nod your head forward (downward) on this horizontal axis. Again hold this position and move your fingers to your nose and nape so the chin swings right. Are you now looking toward the ground on the right with your right ear tilted toward your right shoulder? Can you reverse the order? Can you come to the same point using a different order?

Now repeat each of these rotations moving your eyes first so they draw your head through each of the turns. That is, let your eyes lead your head up and down, then tilting to the left and right, and then rotating to the left and right. Then feel what it is like to do the movement with eyes and head moving precisely at the same time. Notice how different this feels. Which (if either) makes for a smoother movement?

Extra challenge: Consider that your eyes are also small globes with the same axes and planes as your head and your body. You could repeat all the above, simply thinking of the direction of where the axis of rotation might be for your eyes to move in a forward/backward, clockwise/counterclockwise, or horizontal left/right arc. If you can find smooth, slow, small arcs in all these directions, then return to the "wee challenge" and you might be surprised at the difference.

These are simple movements we do all the time, but paying attention to the exactness can make them challenging. Once you have done this process, do you feel different in any way?

To gather maximum information with our teleceptors, our head must have freedom to rotate on all axes, swinging through large angles and refining to small degrees. To scan smoothly at large angles, we enlist much more of ourselves than the few vertebrae at the top of the neck—but the degrees of freedom in those top vertebrae have a profound influence on our orientation and balance.

A small section of the curving skull base sits atop the cradling atlas (first cervical vertebra), which in turn pivots around the peg-like protrusion from the axis (second cervical vertebra). The cradling atlas allows for a small gliding translation of the head, a more subtle and less frequently accessed movement of the head, but one deeply rooted in our early organization. (For example, this glide is part of the early sucking movements from TIY 1-1, Revisit Sucking and Swallowing (p. 93), though not specifically mentioned.)

It is worth repeating TIY 1-1, attending more closely to the degrees of movement available at the very top of the spine, before the neck must flex, extend, or rotate. Your head will not move far in any direction, but finding the subtle multidirectional shifts wakens this area to greater potential.

Juan is an Achuar man of the Ecuadorian Amazon, and every few days he hunts in the dense forest for his family's protein. Like Indigenous hunters everywhere, he has learned to maintain a calm stillness to gather information from his surroundings. His observing stillness is without tension. His head can smoothly tilt and rotate to detect the faint trails of scent, or the small rufflings of movement in the vast tree canopy above him. His head and torso can easily follow the curiosity of his eyes without shifting his balance. The body gives few clues about which direction he will set off in.

If Juan lived his life in a city, he would not have similar encouragement to use all his scanning potential regularly. Many hours facing forward to computer and television screens, in cars or at desks, surrounded by unchallenging sources of sound, buildings that hem in our vision, buffer most of us from the need to move our heads in a diverse range. This restriction of our movement range is implicated in the chronic neck, shoulder, and even vision issues that plague many urban dwellers. Here is a little refresher of your potential.

Try It Yourself 5-2:
Coordinate your eyes, head, and shoulders

Sit comfortably on a firm surface. Look up then down a few times, noticing the range and ease of your movements.

Now turn left then right a few times. Turn slowly enough to notice exactly what turns first. Is it your eyes? What is the timing between your eyes, head, neck, and shoulders as they all engage in the action? The independence of the eyes, often overlooked, is an important element in this TIY, for reasons that should become clearer as we go further.

Now try these seven different combinations of turning around the vertical axis.

1. Eyes, head, and shoulders together to the right.
2. Eyes and head to right, shoulders to left.
3. Eyes and shoulders to right, head to left.
4. Head and shoulders to right, eyes to left.
5. Head to right, shoulders and eyes to left.
6. Eyes to right, shoulders and head to left.
7. Shoulders to right, head and eyes to left.

Repeat the same combinations using opposite sides.

Try all of these several times, slowly enough to notice whether you are doing what you think you are. Are you doing simple rotation around the vertical axis, or are you tilting your head, your shoulders, or even your eyes unnecessarily?

Which combinations feel usual, comfortable, and which feel a bit odd or foreign? These sensations are guideposts to your habits.

Take your time. Soften. Be interested in the process rather than the goal. Be especially interested in the beginning of the movement—that will determine what you do.

Return to simply turning left and right. Is it different? How? How much more of you is involved? Then look up and down again—has this changed, even though we did not work directly with those directions? If there is a change, is it an improvement? In what way? How did your brain generalize this quality of involvement to other movements?

Eyes as Coordinators

As a young woman, Sue had been desperate to get her driver's license. The one thing she hadn't practiced was night driving, but because she had done everything else, she didn't think she needed to worry too much. Her cousin Gus disagreed, so out they went in his old car to a very quiet suburb after dark. Sue was driving well, until there was oncoming traffic. Three times Gus had to quickly correct her steering, before he asked her to pull over to the side of the road. "So where are you looking when a car is coming?" he asked her. "At that car of course," she replied, as if it was a dumb question. "Well every time you look at an oncoming car, our car starts heading toward it! So where do you think you should look?"

This shocked Sue and jogged an old memory of learning to ride a bike. She had constantly ridden into poles and holes until she had learned to keep her eyes on the path she wanted to follow, and not on the obstacle she wanted to avoid. Now it appeared she had fallen into the old habit of looking where she didn't want to go—the oncoming traffic. She had to make a concerted effort to look at the very center of the lane ahead of her. Sue did get the hang of night driving and did get her license. She has continued to notice how often in life people are coached to keep their eye on the ball, or the target, or the finish line, or the prize. The role of the eyes in coordinating muscles for movement has become an abiding interest for her, influencing her choices in further studies.

Of course we can only coordinate that which is ready to cooperate. No leader can guide a team if the members are not willing or able to work together. The microcosm of our own bodies is no different.

Connecting Through the Spine

Lao is a taxi driver. Unfortunately for Lao and his livelihood, he broke several ribs while partying with some friends. When he got back to his cab after weeks of recovery, he found he couldn't turn his head easily to change lanes, reverse, or talk to passengers. Even with rearview mirrors and a rear cam to assist, the limited movement made him tense and anxious in traffic. After only one shift he was in enormous pain.

Lao's grandmother, who had recently migrated to join his family, had quite a reputation as a village healer. Reluctantly Lao asked his sharp-tongued elder for help. She moved him around a bit, prodded and leaned heavily into tightly held muscles, causing Lao to yelp, but also enabling him to take fuller and deeper breaths than he had since the accident. At the end he felt remarkably free and comfortable. He thanked his grandmother and was about to escape her room when she said, "No, bring another chair." Concerned about what was in store for him now, Lao reluctantly obeyed. "Sit here, hold that like a steering wheel," she said, indicating the back of the second chair. "Now look back." He turned, as he had been turning all day in the car, with his shoulders and ribs unmoving while his head rotated less than 45 degrees and then stopped. "Now turn the other way." Again Lao turned but this time managed even fewer degrees. "Hmm, stupid," she grunted, running her fingers up and down his spine. Then, most disturbingly for Lao, she prodded one bony finger into his tailbone, saying, "Turning starts here, not here," as a second bony finger jabbed the base of his neck.

For the next few minutes she placed her sharp fingers at different points of Lao's spine and made him turn his head from that point. Then she did the same to get him bowing his head forward and back and to either side. "Move your head like juggling a plate on a long bamboo stick—from here!" One last time she prodded his tailbone. Lao had the message, loud and clear. His next driving shift changed from an endurance test to an adventure in how many opportunities he could find to turn and tilt his head from different parts of himself, right down to his ankles. The way Lao moves as he drives has changed forever.

We've come to the spine: the central bony structure connecting the head and the pelvis, or separating the head and the pelvis, depending on your perspective. There are many ways to think and talk about the spine other than neck, back, and lower back. Lao's grandmother refers to it as a juggler's stick. We could also liken it to a chain, a long spring, or even an axle. The analogies can provide important clues for how we think about the spine and how we move.

Try It Yourself 5-3:
Imagine your spine

Before continuing, take a moment to consider your image of your own spine.

If you were going to make a clay model of your spine, what might it look like? Do you have a strong image of its three-dimensional shape?

The grandmother wanted Lao to think of his spine as a long flexible stick supporting the weight of a turning head, but with the flexibility to respond as the arms turn the steering wheel or the legs shift across accelerator and brake pedals.

Load-bearing and flexible are in a trade-off relationship. The greater the force we are opposing, or the more strength we wish to exert, the less deviation we want in our systems. (We will talk about this more in OP7 when we deal with pressure, but for now we are looking at images of the spine.) For a weightlifter, during a lift the image of a very flexible spine would be disastrous. Security for a massive lift comes from a firm, column-like connection of pelvis to head, through which the forces can be transmitted directly.

At the other end of the spectrum is the gymnast, who twists, leaps, and progresses through all planes and axes of movement facilitated by the push and pull of long, adaptable limbs. The only load we expect gymnasts to work with is their body mass. The chain or spring analogies work better for this picture of the spine's involvement.

The small increments of movement between our vertebrae connect head to pelvis with a chain-like ability to twist, bend, and pull. When a spine is drawn to its full length by the head or the pelvis, greatest flexibility with least energy expenditure is available.

Our primate cousins, when swinging and leaping through trees, use the pulling and rotating forces available through their long spines to facilitate leaps, spirals, and virtual flight through the air with grace and speed. We may not swing from branches, but each time we take a step our head, shoulders, and swinging arms can create small tugs in changing angles, encouraging length in our long, chain-like spine.

The other way to look at a gymnast's spine is as a sequence of springs. With four long vertical curves and small, gel-like discs between each vertebra, our spines are like a sophisticated series of springs that absorb the shock of rapid compression and rebound that force with every step. The same idea of a long curve as a spring was behind the blade prosthetics designed for amputee runners.

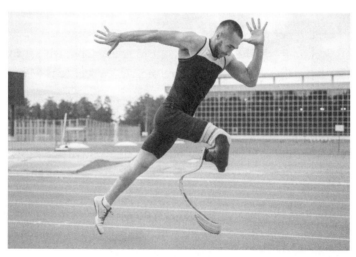

FIGURE 35: Spring-blade-style prosthetic

Finally, there is the spine as a pliable shaft or axle around which elements can rotate. The head can rotate independently of the turning shoulder girdle that likewise can be independent of the pelvic rotation. (This is the rotation explored in TIY 5-1: Find the Axes of Rotation for Your Head, p. 90.) Think of the freestyle swimmer moving through water. The head can lead like an arrow or turn to breathe, as the shoulder girdle rotates to raise one arm and then the other, and the pelvis responds with a different turning rhythm to the alternately kicking feet.

Try It Yourself 5-4:
Re-imagine your spine

This is a very simple walking exercise. Please feel free to take it further, into other positions, paces, or activities if it captures your interest. We have made only a few suggestions for each, which you may well be able to expand.

Walk as if your spine is a solid rod (the proverbial broomstick). What does that do to the sensation of your shoulders and the swing of your arms? What does the world look like when you have a rod for a spine?

Walk as if your spine is a long bamboo stick, able to bend and flex while your head stays central over your pelvis. Does this influence how you feel or see your environment? Does it change the weight on your feet?

Pause for a moment, just to walk without an image in mind before you try the next step.

Walk as if your spine was a chain. How would that influence what you could do, or even what you might like to do? As you walk, does this remind you of anyone you have seen?

Now think of your spine as a spring. As you land on each foot, is there a moment of compression then rebound in any part of your spine? We talk about people walking with a spring in their step—what does a spring in your spine do for your emotional state?

Again pause to stand still, and notice what your spine really feels like to you. You may never have considered this question before, but search it out in your sensations and feelings as much as your thinking.

Finally, take a walk thinking about your spine as a central shaft for the rotating girdles of your pelvis and shoulders, and your head.

Walking now, with no specific image in mind, how do you feel? How is the weight of your walking? Your perception of your own dimensions? The freedom of your head, and the sense of your pelvis?

Rods, chains, springs, and shafts are all images to help feel your spine in movement. But what about actually feeling your spine in its three dimensions? This, of course, presents difficulties. The bulk of the spine faces inward and is protected from touch by impenetrable layers of muscle. If you lie on the floor, press your back against a wall, or have a friend run a hand down your central back, you will feel at least some of those knobby protrusions—the spinal processes. If you are patient, restful, and careful you may even be able to feel some of the transverse processes (the protrusions to the side) in your neck. The largest, sturdiest parts of our spine are beyond our reach, except with our mind's eye. Having a three-dimensional internal sense of the spine can be a profound experience, especially for those who have believed themselves weak, or conceived of their spines as fragile. The solid vertebrae—those stackable blocks of the spine through which forces pass—reach deep into our bodies. The front line of the vertebral body comes very close to our central plumb line at the inmost parts of our lumbar and neck curves.

Try It Yourself 5-5:
Map your spine in line with reality

In TIY 5-3: Imagine Your Own Spine (p. 97), you built a mental map of your spine. Below are pictures of vertebrae and the full spine. How different are these from your own image?

Take a few moments to contemplate each image of the vertebrae below, then "place" them inside your own body.

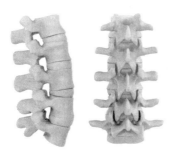 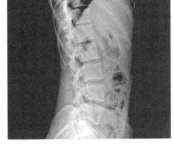

FIGURE 36: Lumbar vertebrae   FIGURE 37: Spine within body

Does having this image change your sensation of support? Or maybe even the experience of sitting right now?

Distributing Forces Across the Whole Spine

We get into difficulties when forces cannot be transmitted directly and sequentially, vertebra to vertebra, through the spine. Physical injury, nerve or neurological damage, trauma of any kind, and of course habitual patterns of use can all interrupt the path of easy transmission and movement along the vertebral chain. For Lao, several weeks of contracting muscles to protect his damaged ribs had left him with a habit of preventing movement through his central (thoracic) spine. Spring, rotation, and sequential pull are limited when segments of the spine rigidify, and other areas must overcompensate. Pain is most likely to occur in overcompensating and hypermobile regions rather than in the immobile sections, erroneously leading people to believe they need to move less rather than distribute movement across more of themselves.

With all this talk of force, it may seem counterintuitive that an extremely effective method for people to free their own spines is to attend to their breathing. Spending time allowing the gentle, unforced flow of breath to gradually reach deeper and wider through the torso can invite even the most consistently and tightly held contractions to finally release. Freedom in length, width, and depth of the torso makes all dimensions available for the spine to respond as needed.

Your Drive: The Pelvis

Finally, we have arrived at the base that supports the torso and head.

The beautiful, undulating belly dancer epitomizes the responsive torso driven by the pelvis. Her gyrating movements, generated from the pelvis, reach all the way to toes, fingers, and head. So too the spiraling launches of the shot put thrower, the wood-shaving sweeps of the carpenter, and even ninety-six-year-old Gianni rising and walking away from his milk crate unaided: they all rely on the same pelvic power.

The results of an effectively moving pelvis distribute through the body, obscuring the source. Commentators praise the knockout punches of a boxer, drawing our attention to the arms and upper torso, sometimes the dancing feet, but few mention the powerful torque from a mobile pelvis that drives both.

All the largest muscles of the body attach at the pelvis, making it the center of our strength and speed. Any restriction of direction or range, at any joint of the pelvis, interferes with the function of those large muscles. To limit the lengthening or shortening capacity of a muscle diminishes the force it can output. Mechanically this is the connection between joint freedom and power. But while the mechanical perspective is important, it is woefully insufficient to explain the global impact of pelvic function in our lives.

For a baby, self-propulsion begins with coordinating the large muscles sufficiently to turn its pelvis. Using the pelvis to roll from back to front (and vice versa) is our very first way of traversing space independently. With that simple roll, the world becomes a more reachable place.

The pelvis remains a region of mystery for most. Even the labeling of the pelvis confuses. To begin with, the word **pelvis** describes a region of our lower torso but is also the collective name for the bones that bound that region.

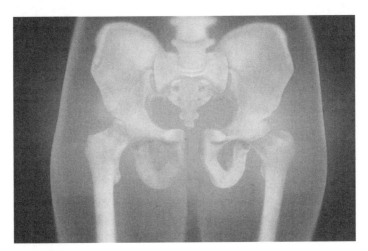

FIGURE 38: Pelvis—from the front

Pelvis and **hips** can be, but are not necessarily, interchangeable. Hip is a rather overworked little word. If a dressmaker or tailor takes a hip measurement, they will measure the widest area of your lower torso, basically where the trunk meets the legs. If you feel your side at this point, you find a large, roundish bony shape. Many mistakenly think of this as the hip bone, but it is part of the "thigh bone" (femur), called the "greater trochanter." Alternatively, any child knows that putting your hands on your hips means to place them on the bony ledges below the waist (the iliac crests).

Yet when a surgeon mentions hip replacement, it is the ball-and-socket joint where the femur meets the pelvis, deep in the groin area, that is the subject.

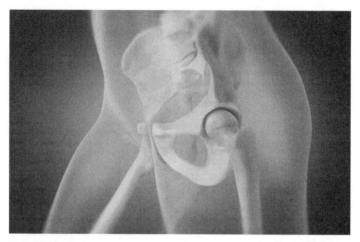

FIGURE 39: Pelvis—from the side

When a man brought up putting his "hands on hips" is told to bend from the hips to touch his toes, where will he attempt to bend from? Most likely not that joint deep in the groin area, which is what the instruction means. How does a woman who thinks her hips are the greater trochanters interpret standing with her feet "hip-width" apart? Her base of support will be much wider than if she thinks of the ball-and-socket joint.

To avoid such confusions, we use **hip** to mean only the ball-and-socket joint where femur and pelvis meet, and **pelvis** rather more generally, to mean both the region and the collection of bones that forms the base of the torso. We recommend that you familiarize yourself with your pelvis in a practical way, investigating its curving bony forms through touch and movement.

Try It Yourself 5-6:
Explore the pelvis

Sit on a firm surface. Are you able to feel the two bones that you now sit on? They are not as wide apart as many think. (Have you noticed saddles on racing bicycles? Although they are narrow, they are still wide enough to support both sit bones.) Lift the right side of your pelvis so you can slide your right hand beneath, palm up. When you settle your pelvis back down, can you feel the sit bone on top of your right hand? If not, keep moving your hand until you can feel this bone resting on your fingers. You should be able to roll backward and forward on the right side, over your hand, feeling slightly different angles and areas of the sit bone coming into contact. Can you get a sense of your entire pelvis moving backward and forward as you do this?

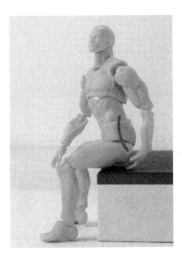 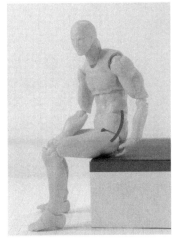

FIGURE 40: Sit bone (ischial tuberosity)—rolling forward over hand

FIGURE 41: Sit bone (ischial tuberosity)—rolling backward over hand

When you have satisfied your curiosity, remove your hand, sit "flat" on the surface again, and see how this feels. For many it will feel as if you are sitting further down on the right, as if there is a dip in the seat on that side.

This time sit with your knees wide and place your right hand underneath the right sit bone by reaching from inside the right leg. From this position, as you feel for the path of the bone forward and upward you will find layers of strong muscles impede your direct contact with the bone. With a little patience you can still track the firmness of the bone lying beneath. You can feel towards your midline, where the pubic bone becomes a narrow bridge connecting left and right halves of the pelvis. Moving away from the bridge to the right you can follow the sweep all the way up to the "ledges" (iliac crests) we can place our hands on. There are no muscles going over the bones at this upper edge, so it is very easy to make contact, until you continue your reach around the back to where the pelvis meets the spine. Again ligament and muscle layers crisscross this joining region, but feel downward at the center of your back and you will find the gently curving sacrum that leads down between the buttocks to the inward-tilting tailbone.

Sit still for a moment and now experience your sense of your pelvis on the right—is there a difference between right and left?

You have now explored the dimensions of your pelvis on the right. Try the same on the left, until you have defined the pelvic outline with your hands.

Sit quietly and see if it is now easier to sense your pelvis, without your hands. Once you have felt the external surface, you can begin to sense out the bowl-like interior of the pelvis using a combination of your mind's eye, proprioceptors, and interoceptors.

Roll a little forward and backward on your sit bones and see if you can mentally track the path of the iliac crests as you roll, then track the path of your tailbone and sacrum as you roll. Can you hold a three-dimensional image of your pelvis as you are rolling forward and back?

Try tilting your pelvis left and right, still holding the three-dimensional image. Can you rotate so one side of the pelvis comes forward and then the other, still holding the three-dimensional image? As you stand up, can you track the movement of your pelvis, and which axes of rotation are most involved?

Pause to reflect—do any elements of standing or walking feel different after doing this exploration?

This exercise informs your self-image in a very practical way, for without a pelvis in your self-image, your platform for power and support is missing.

Pelvis in Action

If nowhere else, most adults have come across some information on the pelvis as the base of power in reference to lifting. Though the word "pelvis" may be absent, there is plenty of information about lifting with the legs, the buttocks, backside, and core, all referring to the pelvic region or the large muscles attached to the pelvis. Back-care classes, workplace health and safety manuals, even weight rooms in gyms constantly reinforce the message we seem to collectively forget. That is—to lift weight, we need to bring the pelvis as close to the load as possible, with the head oriented in the direction we wish to move (up) and the spine prepared for an upward push through feet, legs, and pelvis. Yet when a region is not clear in our self-image, or our sensation, external messages like these are easily forgotten. Waiting rooms for doctors and therapists still fill with people who have bent over the top of heavy loads and attempted to lift them by pulling with arms and upper torso, leading to disastrous results for the spine. Any wild animal so careless with its well-being would perish.

Like every other part of us, the pelvis and its attachments and joints are shaped by our habitual use, misuse, or disuse. As the central juncture for receiving and transmitting forces through our system, it needs to be continuously adaptable to the requirements of our position and activity. When our pelvic region is engaged effectively, movement of our head and limbs feel light, and full range is available at our joints. In other words, the benefits of a responsive, weight-bearing, force-generating pelvis are felt throughout the system. On the flip side, poor use of our pelvic structure will show up diversely, but especially at major stress points like knees, feet, shoulders, or neck.

Stef has always loved being active, but she was plagued by plantar fasciitis (sharp pain at the heel and along the sole of the foot) for nearly a year. She could no longer run, walking had lost its pleasure, and her first step each morning caused pain. There were many treatments offered and tried—exercises, anti-inflammatory drugs, massage, ice and heat protocols, shoe inserts . . . Some gave her short-term relief, but improvements from the treatments never seemed to last. After ten months of trying, surgery was suggested. She wasn't keen, and she discussed this option with her close friend Bel. Bel was an avid gardener, and there were few situations she didn't find a gardening analogy for. "You know," said Bel, "we might all be looking in the wrong place. Sometimes I turn on a sprinkler but hardly any water comes out. I can check it, make sure it's not blocked or broken, but usually the answer is not where I first notice the problem. Usually it's back up the line where there is a twist or split in the hose that I haven't noticed. So just because the pain is in your foot doesn't mean that's where the real issue is." Before committing to surgery on her foot, Stef decided to find someone to help her look "up the line."

For Stef the turning point came when she began to address how she walked, not just how her foot contacted the ground. She began to look at how her stride was initiated through her lower torso.

All of us have small asymmetries in our pelvis and spine. We grow up doing asymmetrical actions like preferring one leg to kick and one to stabilize, one leg to turn around, one side to kneel on. This is a healthy and normal occurrence for developing proficiency. If we use a good diversity of movements, the asymmetrical use is balanced out. But if we don't have adequate variety, we tend to reinforce holding patterns that limit joint freedom. These patterns have a bearing on how we walk, particularly how we transfer the weight of our torso across our feet to progress forward.

When Stef slowed down her walk, she could begin to feel how, in parts of the transfer, her pelvis and lower spine stiffened, which caused her foot to "grasp" at the ground. It was subtle, but as she trained her attention on the initiation of each step, she was able to detect the difference between gliding the pelvis forward in continuous motion and inhibiting some of the pelvic mobility. She found many opportunities across her days to experiment with the continuous movement of her pelvis, gradually adding more directions of movement. At some point the plantar fasciitis simply disappeared. She had noticed it diminish from chronic to intermittent, then one day she noticed nothing—the pain had simply not occurred. Finally, with care, she has returned to the running she loves, with the bonus that her gait also feels freer and lighter than before.

Pelvic strength and adaptability impact every sphere of human action.

The same axes of rotation that we explored for the head are available for the pelvis. Because the pelvis is so central to power and balance, developing an internal, three-dimensional sense of its structure in action can improve all aspects of your movement.

The following TIY is an active way to build awareness of the rotations of the pelvis. Many cultures have ways to liberate the pelvis for speed, mobility, and power. For example, Polynesian dancers use foliage-laden "hip" bands and belly dancers use coin-weighted scarves not just as costumes but to focus their attention on pelvic movement during practice.

Try It Yourself 5-7:
Explore three dimensions, with a broomstick

Take a long stick, such as a broom handle, and place it horizontally against your body, along the top of your pubic bone. The stick will now be passing across the region of your hip joints. Anchor your hands against your pelvis at the sides, so you can feel the motion of the pelvis while still holding the stick. Now the stick can magnify the movements of the pelvis.

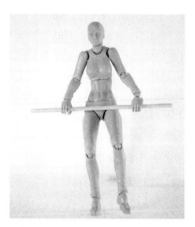

FIGURE 42: Lightening one foot—
horizontal stick at front of pelvis

Slowly begin to lighten one foot from the ground, preparing to step forward but not yet taking a step. Repeat this movement a few times, and notice what happens at the stick (pelvis) for your foot to lighten. Does it translate sideways across the standing leg? Does it tilt up or down over the about-to-move leg? The movement will be very different depending on where your feet are in relation to your hip joints. Are they directly beneath the joints? Wider? Or are you standing with feet together? Try a few different positions of your feet, and see what difference that makes to the initial direction of movement in your pelvis and the simplicity of shifting weight from one foot to the other.

Step forward with one foot. Notice one side of the stick moves forward. As you begin to lift your heel to step forward, what happens to the stick on that side? Does it tilt up and down, or forward and back?

Continue to play with stepping forward and backward, noticing the shapes the ends of the stick draw in the air. Do they make circles, ellipses, figure eights, or odd, unnameable shapes? How do you need to move with your spine and head to change the shape? Does one side make a larger shape than the other?

Don't get trapped in thinking there is an ideal shape you should make as you walk forward or backward. Just notice what's happening, and play with how you can change and increase or decrease the fullness of the shapes. Curiosity and playfulness will help more than idealism.

If you can begin to match the feeling of the moving pelvis to the visual aid of the stick moving, you can begin to build a three-dimensional image of the pelvic action. To increase the experience of dimension, you could place the stick behind you, sitting horizontally against the sacrum with your fists against the back of your pelvis.

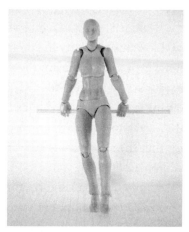

FIGURE 43: Lightening one foot—
horizontal stick at rear of pelvis

Give yourself time, because building this picture in your mind's eye is something your brain needs time and multiple repetitions over days, not minutes, to achieve. Be aware of the common tendency to hold the head still with glazed, fixed eyes when asked to pay attention while moving. Counter it by bringing your attention up every now and then to ensure your head and neck are free, responding to the movement of pelvis and spine, so that movement can travel the length of your body.

Put the stick down and take a few steps forward and backward. Can you still track the motion that each side of your pelvis makes as you step? To help your brain develop a better map of this region, you could keep the stick handy, so you can pick it up and play with it a few times a day for several days.

Pelvis as Support

Not only power but also finesse starts with effective use of the pelvis. Light arms, delicate manipulations, freedom through the neck and shoulders all require the anchoring, strong work of support to be done by the pelvis and legs. Violinists, painters, computer operators, woodworkers, and so on all have this necessity in common.

Paul is a shy young man with a dream. He wants to be a kayak champion. For the most part he has self-trained, picking up tips from the internet and working hard in his neighbor's home gym when he can. Paul believes the secret to kayaking lay in developing his arms and chest. He reasons that the stronger his arms, the more powerfully he can draw his paddle through the water. So he has worked hard on his triceps, biceps, deltoids, "traps," and anything else the internet gurus promote for upper-body strength. He started doing quite well in competitions, but every few months he would injure a shoulder or develop pain in his neck that slowed his training frustratingly.

When his neighbor moved away, Paul had to join a commercial gym. He found himself among other enthusiasts with diverse aspirations and perspectives. It was a random conversation comparing riding horses to shooting rapids that, for the first time, made him question the role of his lower torso when kayaking. With more exploration and information, his whole training regimen turned upside down. As he has increased his lower-body strength and the connection to his base of support, he has discovered he no longer feels great effort in his arms as he paddles. His arms are now light and responsive to the water in a way he had never imagined. His consistent neck and shoulder injuries have disappeared.

Paul discovered that his legs cannot sit flaccidly on the bottom of a kayak if he wishes to generate the torque force through his torso that turns the paddle with ease. Kayaking, as Paul found, is a whole-body sport.

Try It Yourself 5-8:
Coordinate your pelvis, spine, and head

Sit on a chair with a firm seat, close enough to a table so you can lean forward, resting your elbows and forearms in a manner that can support you lightly.

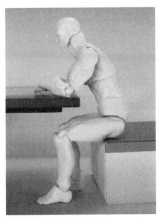

FIGURE 44: Seated—supported on forearms

Look up, allowing your eyes and head to move as you also roll forward on your pelvis. Notice that this makes a shallow C curve of your spine—longer on the front, shorter on the back.

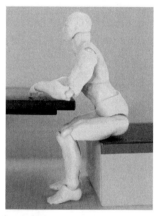

FIGURE 45: Seated—pelvis rolled forward to create spinal C curve

Look down and roll backward on your pelvis, reversing the C curve so it is longer on the back, shorter on the front.

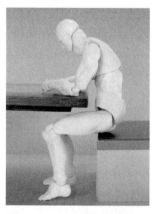

FIGURE 46: Seated—pelvis rolled backward to reverse spinal C curve

Gently repeat these two directions until you can spread your attention to include pelvis, spine, and head fluidly.

In your present position you are supported by your arms, pelvis, and legs. Now continue to move between the two C curves while you spread your attention to the shoulder and hip joints. Can you feel how their freedom is important in enabling the spine to curve and the limbs to support?

Now try a new angle—a diagonal.

Look up to your right as you roll your pelvis forward to the right. Your weight moves predominantly over your right sit bone and you find you are getting longer on the right side and front, shorter on left side and back.

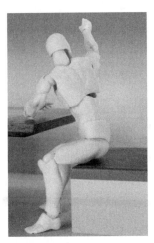

FIGURE 47: Looking and reaching up to the right as weight moves to right sit bone

Release your right arm and reach up to the right as you look there. Smoothly change direction to take your eyes and right hand down toward the left foot. Allow your weight to roll to the left and back of the pelvis as you reach down to the inside of the left foot, following with your eyes, head, and upper torso. Now that the arm is involved, can you still find the asymmetrical roll of weight on your pelvis?

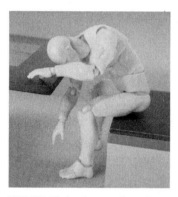

FIGURE 48: Looking and reaching down to the left as weight moves to left sit bone

Reverse the action, so you take your hand and eyes from the left foot in a smooth arc up to the top-right corner again. Can you feel the roll of your pelvis from back left, through the center, to forward right as you do this?

Take your time and stay in a very small range so your attention can match the action with your sensations. You are combining lengthening on the right side and front with shortening on the left side and back. You will have done this many times in your life, but probably not with the attention you are using now, so it can be confusing.

You might like to play with this on the opposite diagonal, using the left hand to reach up to the left as your head and eyes follow it, and so on. Or you might like to skip to the next bit, for the moment.

Feel the difference with these combinations if you initiate the movement from your pelvis, your head, or your eyes. Which allows for greater ease? Which feels like the action incorporates more of you?

Do some of these combinations feel more usual to you than others?

Return to normal sitting, no longer leaning on your arms. By exploring these different shapes/trajectories and finding different ways to relate the movement of your pelvis and head, what has happened to your sense of ease in sitting? Do you feel more supported? Do you have a different sense of the space both inside you and around you? How easily could you move in different directions to stand and do something?

Parts of the Whole

There is no end of ways we can divide up the body into anatomical parts, physiological systems, regions of function or form, and so on. Each way brings its own insights and its own limitations. For the most part, the separation and naming of parts serves us best to understand a still or inert body. In action, the labeling makes less sense and can even impede easy, effortless movement. For instance, turning the head with ease involves musculoskeletal adjustment all the way to the pelvis, and even the feet if we are standing. As we grow, however, we separate the head from the body in language. This separates the head in thought and can unintentionally flow through to restricting action. Many adults isolate the action of turning to their head and neck, thereby chronically limiting range and ease.

The challenge is to go beyond the separation and rediscover the relationship of parts to the whole. All the stories in this chapter have been about rediscovering relationship—Lao learning how his ribs and tailbone were involved in freeing his head to turn; Paul finding that strengthening his pelvic region and legs freed his shoulders and lightened his arms while increasing his paddling power; and Stef unearthing the connection between an immobile section of her spine and the plantar fasciitis that had confounded her.

OP6

POWER IS CENTRAL AND PRECISION PERIPHERAL

Strength and force come from the center, while direction and accuracy come from the extremities

LEE TRAVELS AND WRITES for a living, but on her last trip she witnessed something that she found difficult to capture in words. It was a young woman who, without exchanging a word, had changed the way Lee thought about human capacity. She'd seen her in the dining room of a bed-and-breakfast, sitting in a wheelchair, holding her morning coffee with her foot. The young woman calmly raised the mug to her mouth, sipped, then placed it back on the table. Lee was transfixed. This woman had no arms, but was nonchalantly sipping coffee and eating toast using her foot, while chatting with a companion. Embarrassed by her own gaping, Lee forced herself to look away, fetch a breakfast, then deliberately sit where she could not stare. The next time she saw her, the young woman was leaving. The same foot that had so expertly grasped the coffee mug was now on the ground, in a soft-soled shoe, and pushing her backward in the wheelchair. Her other leg appeared to be amputated above the knee.

Lee went back to her room, sat on her bed, and tried to bring her foot to her mouth. Without using her hands to catch and pull her foot it was completely impossible. Even with her hands it was extremely difficult. She couldn't imagine how her foot might grasp a coffee cup while her leg traveled to her mouth with no arms. Lee understood necessity would have been the young woman's teacher, but the mere idea that this was a human capacity dormant in all of us was bewildering to her.

By our teen years, most of us have a solid concept of how our body parts are to be used. Our cultures, environments, and personal histories limit our repertoires and, barring exceptional events, they remain unchallenged. A small percentage of people escape these limitations by pursuing physically challenging interests, but for the most part we unwittingly accept a meager range of what is possible, relegating all else to impossible and quite literally unthinkable.

You may never need to use your foot to drink your coffee, but if your toes and foot were capable of grasping a handle, your leg able to smoothly lift and bring your foot toward your mouth, your hip joint and spine capable of responding to the demand of this lift, and your central nervous system could coordinate all this without spilling hot coffee, then what else might your toes, feet, legs, spine—you—be capable of?

In anatomical language, what we are talking about is the relationship between proximal and distal. **Proximal** means nearest the center of mass ("in proximity"); **distal** means away from the center of mass ("distant"). These are relative terms. The shoulder is proximal when compared to the hand, but the wrist is proximal when compared to fingers. Relative to just about every other part of our bodies, the pelvis is proximal and our fingers and toes (digits) are distal.

We are going to keep returning to this story, so rather than continually saying "the young woman," let's call her Ada. Not only could Ada bring her leg past her center with great precision, she also knew how to push power from her center to her foot to propel her wheelchair. This chapter is about the relationship between our extremities and our center that Ada exemplified. We will explore how our center can empower delicate work at our extremities, and our extremities provide direction for our center.

Two Ends of an Action

For most actions, our attention fixes on our distal parts, which move through space more than our proximal parts. We extend an arm out to pick up a glass and bring it all the way back to our torso and head to take a sip. Or do we? Is this only an action of the arm, or are the proximal parts involved as more than an anchor point? For any person who has experienced joint pain, this principle may be enormously important.

At a musculoskeletal level, we move because our muscles are either contracting or releasing. When a muscle contracts, the pulling force at both ends is the same, just like elastic. If you connect two equivalent objects with elastic, hold them apart, then release the objects simultaneously, they will spring back together equally. The elastic, like our muscles, pulls both with the same force. If, however, one object is heavier, then the lighter object will move further than the heavy one, even though the elastic is still pulling both ends equally. When one object is disproportionally heavy, extremely stable, or fixed in some way, the reciprocal pull is not extinguished, but it becomes imperceptible. Sir Isaac Newton spoke of the pulling force of gravity in the same way: "If matter thus draws matter, it must be proportion of its quantity. Therefore, the apple draws the Earth, as well as the Earth draws the apple."[1]

---

[1] Quoted in William Stukeley's 1752 memoir of Sir Isaac Newton.

In the human body, some parts obviously have greater mass, but the dynamic nature of our balance should mean that both ends of a contracting muscle are pulled toward each other, even though the distance traveled differs.

Try It Yourself 6-1:
Lift with attention

Sit at a table with a mug, glass, or drink bottle in front of you.

Reach out with your hand and lift the drink just a little. When you lift does your shoulder or your torso come forward slightly?

Deliberately keep your torso absolutely still as you again lift the drink. Can you feel that to fix your torso in space you must engage some muscles in the torso—maybe not heavily, but contracting nevertheless? You may even feel the sit bone on the "active" side push into the seat a little. However, if this is your habitual way to lift an object, you may feel none of those things because they are so automatic—therefore try what might be non-habitual.

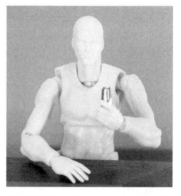

FIGURE 49: Lifting object with still torso

Place a finger of your other hand at the top of your sternum (breast bone), and next time you lift your drink in the direction of your mouth, allow the sternum to slightly turn and move toward the lifting object. Of course allow your head and eyes to also respond with the sternum. Can you feel your shoulders turning and moving gently, slightly forward, as you lift the drink toward your mouth? Can you lift the drink higher more easily?

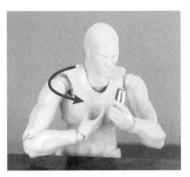

FIGURE 50: Lifting as sternum, head, and eyes turn toward object

Next time you are about to lift, begin by preemptively turning your shoulders and torso toward the object, and notice if it now moves toward you even faster and lighter.

Keep holding the drink as it rests back on the table, and now bring your sternum to the object—that is, bring the center of yourself toward your distal part. Notice the change in efficiency and effort when we move the greater to the lesser parts.

Try alternating between lifting with a fixed torso and lifting while allowing both ends to respond toward each other. See if you can feel the difference in the experience of effort, the sensation in your shoulder, or maybe in your freedom of breath.

Go back to the simplicity of lifting your drink toward your mouth and see how much of yourself can easily cooperate in this action.

Although we commonly think and speak as if actions are isolated to specific regions of the body, in reality this is rare. The previous TIY invites you to experience the cooperative movement that takes place in a well-performed action. Lifting one arm changes the balance of the entire body and requires a widespread musculoskeletal response that we are not trained to notice.

When both ends of a contracting muscle can respond appropriately, we are not wasting energy on opposing contractions. More than that, the largest muscles of the torso are now able to cooperatively assist the limbs, making work lighter. For someone with joint pain, such as a frozen shoulder, this distribution of workload without contradictory contraction is very important.

If you are keen on heavier forms of exercise, like workouts at a gym, you can still benefit from this concept. Exercises like push-ups, bicep curls, or squats can be experienced differently once you understand that, like Newton's apple drawing the Earth, each end of a contraction is drawn toward the center even when one end is fixed. For instance, as you lower yourself in a push-up, consider that your hands are pulling back toward your chest as your chest lowers to your hands. Your hands will not lift, but you might experience a surprise lightening. Similarly, squat with the intention to feel that small pull of your feet toward your pelvis as your pelvis is lowered toward your feet. (This is not about lifting your heels, driving the front of your feet more heavily into the floor, but feeling the entirety of both feet drawn toward your pelvis.)

Aesthetics vs. Function

Sadly, for most of us brought up in a Western culture, we were taught from an early age that an upright, unmoving torso signals a respectful attitude for listening and learning, that it is both good posture and aesthetically pleasing. This aesthetic penetrates all manner of places. Orchestral musicians lifting and playing awkward instruments asymmetrically have been required to keep a still torso so as not to distract the audience. Generations of women office workers were taught to sit rigidly in office chairs, as symbols of neat efficiency. To achieve this ideal we must inhibit the efficient use of our global muscles and siphon power away from action to anchoring. At the same time, we are requiring the inverse from local muscles—requiring greater range from small muscles designed only to stabilize. We are working against ourselves.

Culturally we have prioritized an external visual image of orderly posture over an internal sense of flexible strength. Many instances of chronic back pain and repetitive strain injury have their roots in this static concept.

Center and Periphery Working Together

Let's return to Ada for a moment. Lee was transfixed by Ada's ability to smoothly bring her foot to her mouth, leveling the tilt of the coffee mug all the way so no drop was spilled. Such startling, unexpected skills distract us from what makes that movement possible. Just as lifting the arm in the previous TIY changed the balance of the body and required a whole system response, so does Ada's smoothly rising leg emerge from coordination of her whole self.

Here's one way to describe what is happening. Ada's leg needs to feel light enough to lift through a wide arc. You cannot lift a limb that is also being used for support, so she must be in a position where weight can easily shift on her base of support. As the leg lightens, freed of weight-support duty, Ada's toes, feet, and ankles can find the sensitivity to adjust with finesse around the mug. She is now going to make a large asymmetrical movement: sweeping her foot from the table to her mouth. Each moment of that arc changes her center of gravity, requiring continuous readjustment through the torso. Remember that Ada has no arms with which to prop herself. While the powerful global muscles of the torso are lifting her leg, local muscles at the joints of the spine, ribs, shoulder girdle, pelvis, and head must constantly adapt to find dynamic balance. Meanwhile the finesse that orients mouth and mug together in a splash-free encounter comes from the finer muscles of both the foot and the face. Of course, during such a well-organized movement, Ada won't be consciously thinking of any of these elements. She will have a single intention that makes it possible—to take a sip of coffee while she chats with her friend.

Here's a summary: Ada's strength, stability, and dexterity are the result of coordination between conditioned muscles, a balanced mobile bone structure, and a healthy nervous system.

Specialization of Power and Direction

Our most powerful skeletal muscles are central and attached to the pelvis (this was covered in OP5). The more peripheral the muscles, the finer they become, more suited to directing than supplying power. We use proximal power to raise a limb, and distal dexterity to direct action.

A carpenter must use proximal power for the rise and descent of a hammer, but the fine muscles of the forearm and hand must have freedom to adjust the hammer's trajectory to the nail head. Many an apprentice has learned, painfully, that the grasp on the hammer must be light while power is transmitted from the torso.

Try It Yourself 6-2:
Let your foot direct your torso

Sit on a chair or bench and visualize for a moment bringing the sole of your foot toward your mouth. What would the first 5 to 10 percent of that movement entail?

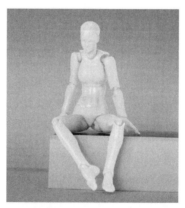

FIGURE 51: Small turn and lift of foot toward mouth

Now do the first 5-10 percent of that journey of foot to mouth. Can you feel, as you turn your foot to lift it in the direction of your mouth, that your knee turns outward? Notice the arc the knee travels as the sole of the foot reorients.

Remember from the previous section that as powerful muscles are lifting the leg—even a short way—something is also happening to the other end of those muscles. What happens in your torso at the very beginning of this lift? Try not to make something happen; just feel what is.

Keep repeating this small 5-10 percent of the movement. Each time you repeat you can make it simpler and lighter.

As you repeat, take your attention further up the leg to the hip joint. Can you feel how, to lift the foot and allow the knee to turn out, the head of the femur (long upper leg bone) must rotate in the hip socket? That rotation changes the entire weight distribution of how you sit. If you stay with this experience for several repetitions, you might feel more deeply how your weight and your pelvis respond to the demand of lifting the leg. If you didn't have your other leg to counterbalance you, how would you have to shift your weight to continue?

If you experience your lower back arching a little forward as you begin to lift your foot, notice the weight of your leg. Do this a few times—as a small movement—then lift your leg but allow your pelvis to sink a little backward as you do. Can you feel the abdominals now engage and the leg become lighter as the spine is allowed to curve backward? Those global abdominal muscles are attached to the pelvis and the front of the rib cage. They flex the torso while the cooperative response from the extensors of the back is to release into length. (If your lower back shortens and arches forward, you have a contradictory response that is making the movement more effortful than needed.)

Does it help if you time this action on an outward breath?

As you continue to notice the pathway of action when you lift the foot, allowing the knee and hip to turn, you might start to notice a demand on your sternum to turn slightly and yield toward the rising foot or the turning knee. Can you find the connection between the outward swinging knee and the yielding of the rib cage?

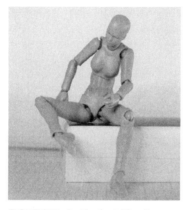

FIGURE 52: As the foot lifts, the knee swings out and the sternum yields toward the foot

As you repeat this last piece of the action, aim to make it softer, lighter, and simpler each time. If your eyes, head, and sternum turn gently toward your foot, you might find the rib cage yields further to the movement, bringing the head toward the foot with no increased effort.

After you have finished this process, stand up and walk around, noticing the difference between the "worked" side and the "unworked" side. Can you notice a difference in length, weight, or stability between the sides? Some people may even feel that one side of the face feels remarkably different after this short experiment.

In OP5 we spoke about the eyes coordinating the torso for action. This last TIY approaches from the opposite end. The proprioceptors in the muscles and joints of the foot and ankle begin a cascade of coordination.

Now that we have drawn attention to the coordination roles of eyes and feet (hands, too, even though we have not included them yet), you will easily recognize that the head is in the same distal relationship to the torso as are our arms and legs. In this sense, you could say the head is like a fifth limb. In OP5, we discussed the necessity for our head to be free to orient and guide the power-generating pelvis. The hands and feet also coordinate and guide, though at a different organizational level.

Freeing the Limbs

Just as our head needs to be free to scan, so our limbs also need freedom if they are to lead actions. Yet limbs also need to bear weight, support us, and transport us. As we've already mentioned, a limb cannot simultaneously support weight and be light enough to lift and direct. We spend many years refining the transition from one role to the other, using foundations laid down in our very first forays into crawling.

In OP1 we looked at weight transfer and dynamic balance. In OP3 we looked at the increasing sophistication of weight-bearing with each stage of the developmental sequence. Though the limbs have been involved in all of these, much of the attention was on the organization through the torso. So let's shift that attention for a moment.

As flexion and extension through the torso have become more coordinated and sophisticated, infants have been progressing onto elbows and knees, then hands and knees, to hands and feet, and finally feet only. The head has become free to orient and limbs intermittently free of weight-bearing to reach, hold, and manipulate. Our limbs become levers to transmit force from the center, while our hands and feet develop dexterity to adjust to the environment.

Using Tools

With sufficient coordination, the objects we originally grasp out of curiosity become tools for manipulation—tools extend our reach into the world and exponentially expand the ways we interact with it. The maturing specialization between proximal and distal becomes increasingly important as our reach extends. Proficiency with tools is a consequence of proficiency in our own movement.

Using tools requires us to become more resourceful in finding points of support so our extremities are free for finesse. To write, both children and adults will rest and slide their wrists or forearms on stable surfaces, thereby supporting their arms while fingers have the freedom and finesse to form letters. On a mouse for a computer we will do the same, allowing arm and mouse to move through space in a supported way, leaving fingers free to click or scroll. Some artists use sticks secured between the canvases and themselves to support their arm's weight while allowing their fingers to lightly guide their brushes. The more precise the activity, the more we will tend to find some movable support close to the action.

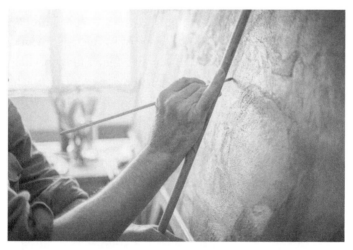

FIGURE 53: Using a mahlstick to support hand for fine brushstrokes

When props or multiple points of support are not an option, we must return to our earliest solutions for distributing weight and decreasing load. Hairdressers, pianists, and others who cannot anchor their wrists or prop their elbows to free their hands must shorten the long levers of their arms by keeping their elbows close to their bodies. Not only do they learn to tuck their elbows close to their torsos, but they adjust heights of stools and tables and length of instruments to minimize the requirement to extend their arms for prolonged times. Their structural support must now come from the shoulder girdle, which in turn is supported from our pelvis, torso, and legs.

Balancing the demands of exertion and accuracy has probably been exercising minds since hunter-gatherer times. Below is an illustration from the seventeenth century of a violinist, famed in his day, showing the two strategies for removing load from his extremities to free their agility—he finds structural support by pressing his elbow into his rib cage, and he shortens the lever by constraining the range of his upper arm's movements on the bowing arm.

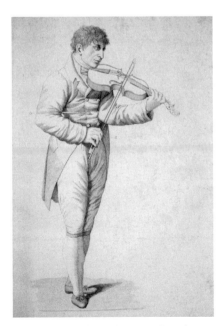

FIGURE 54: Violin technique—Bartolomeo Campagnoli

The upsides of adjusting our environment with props and well-designed tools are extending the time we can be occupied without fatigue and minimizing wear and tear on our joints. The downside is becoming so habituated to an adjusted environment that we decrease the variety of movements in our lives. It is well worth each person's while to strip away all their tools, aids, and props for some time each day to encourage their incredible shape-changing torso to move and be moved by the five limbs.

OP7

PRESSURE ORGANIZES

The demands of internal or external pressure create and test our ability to respond with well-organized movement

BEA IS AN AVERAGE singer, with ambition. Out of curiosity she recently attended a workshop run by a quirky voice coach with a fearsome reputation. Bea had the dubious honor of being first to sing solo in front of the group. As usual when she was reaching for the high notes, both her breath and voice waned into a short, thin thread of sound. She expected a lecture on breath support or tight jaws or another common "fix." Instead she was taken to a table and told to lift the side of it. It wasn't too heavy but required her to adjust her feet and handholds to lift well. The coach watched her, grunted "Good," then asked her to sing the passage with the high notes again—only this time, as she ascended in pitch she was to lift the side of the table. Bea and the onlookers were astounded: her voice sailed strongly through the whole passage, steady, clear, and true. Somehow the lifting task had organized her breathing and singing in a way no focus on parts or mechanisms had ever done. We will unpack the reasons for this as we go forward.

Meeting Pressure with Pressure

You might not easily recognize Bea's story as an issue of organizing pressure. We could have started by returning to the two Graces of OP2, whose responses to the pressure of gravity were shaping their bones. However, Bea's story represents the diverse forms pressures take as we mature. We constantly deal with external physical loads, internal emotional tensions, intellectual and physiological stressors. Recognizing this diversity and the adequacy of our response is an important part of dealing with pressure.

From the moment of conception, our structure has been adapting to these pressures using fluids, membranes, and valves.

Though we may commonly consider the fluids (gases, liquids, and fluidized solids) in our body as the transport system for distributing nutrients, removing waste, and couriering chemical messages, they are so much more. Within every human, in fact every animal, are a series of hydraulic systems that shape and movement are founded upon.[1]

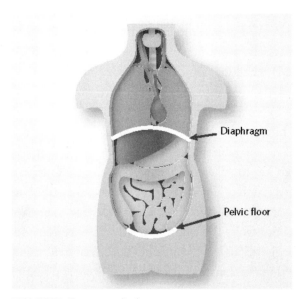

FIGURE 55: Torso as cylinder

---

[1] This is explored in the field of biological fluid dynamics.

Think of the torso as a flexible cylinder with a framework of bones, connective tissue, and muscles. The spine runs from top to bottom, giving vertical support. The circumference is maintained at one end by the ribs and at the other by the pelvis. Though no bones cross the abdominal expanse, we are girdled by powerful global muscles. In standing, the bones of the pelvis bear the load of our flesh- and fluid-filled form.

At each end of the cylinder are a series of valves that allow intake or outlet: the glottis and soft palate at the top, and the sphincters in the pelvic floor, which forms the cylinder's base. Between them we have the diaphragm—the sheet of muscle that separates the abdominal and thoracic cavities. The diaphragm and pelvic floor are the piston equivalents. When the diaphragm contracts, it flattens downward, gently compressing the fluid-filled abdomen and creating a vacuum above that can fill with air—breath. The pelvic floor lifts upward when it contracts. If both the diaphragm and the pelvic floor contract at the same time, the pressure between the two contracting muscles—the intra-abdominal pressure—increases to a strong stabilizing pressure. Simultaneous contraction is, however, only one of the many ways the two muscles might relate. Each contracts or releases in its own timing and intensity to fulfill widely divergent functions—think of laughing, which is a light, rapid contract/release of the diaphragm, while holding a sustained contraction of the pelvic floor as you wait in a queue for the toilet.

The diaphragm, in cooperation with muscles around the ribs, the abdominal walls, the pelvic floor, and the throat, coordinates the flow and pressure of fluids throughout the torso, creating a powerful hydraulic system.

From birth our innate survival movements—sucking, swallowing, breathing, crying, and defecating—begin the coordination of pressure through the torso. As we grow, and the size and sources of load on our system increase, we need a constantly adaptable relationship between the diaphragm and the pelvic floor to adjust intra-abdominal pressure.

To become more aware of abdominal pressure and its phenomenal role in our well-being, we start with muscles.

Strong Muscles May Cover Weakness

We have discussed the distinction between global muscles and local muscles in OP2 and touched on them in OP5 and OP6, but it is worth repeating with a new addition. If a body is well aligned in gravity, the local muscles switch on and support its structure, leaving global muscles to move us through space in shape-changing actions. However, when not well aligned over the base of support, global muscles must take over much of the support system for the structure, diminishing their role in coordinating fluid pressure. The diaphragm and pelvic floor are also harnessed into structural support, which limits their ability to adapt to changing conditions. In this way, breathing and other pressure-related functions are hampered by poor alignment.

Try It Yourself 7-1:
Engage global muscles for support

Sit simply on a firm stool or bench—someplace where you can easily lean back without obstruction.

Place your hands on your lower abdomen.

Begin to slowly lean backward so your head moves behind your center of gravity. As you lean, you will feel large abdominal muscles (beneath your hands) switch on and hold you as you tilt. You do not need to tilt extremely, just until you feel the abdominals firming.

As you tilt, what happens to your breath? Do you feel yourself holding or closing anything in your throat? If you pay careful attention you may feel the abdominal muscles begin to draw your ribs into the contraction, making it more difficult to expand your rib cage for a breath.

Return to upright, notice the abdominals release, and then begin the tilt back again, noticing the relationship between the abdominals switching on and the changing of your breath. Try it a few times so you have time to notice what you do. When you tilt and are no longer centered over your base of support, the large muscles must engage to support you. When you are centered over your base of support, your local muscles can support the head, spine, and pelvic alignment and the larger global muscles can release.

In this TIY, you were moving outside your base of support to experience the large abdominal muscles switching into a strong support pattern. There is no problem doing this in the short term. Long term, however, is a different matter. If our global muscles are used consistently for support, the local muscles whose role is to secure joints, wrapping the spine in a lattice of supple reinforcement, are not effectively used. They begin to weaken.

Lex works on construction sites. During his workday he is constantly transferring loads to locations mechanical devices can't reach. He may be carrying beams on his shoulders, barrowing bags of cement over rough ground, hefting heavy equipment into position to drill, saw, or sand, and so on. He's been working in the building industry for more than twenty years and appears to be strong and well coordinated working with awkward shapes and weights. So it was a huge surprise to Lex and his wife when he started developing severe back pain at home. At work he was virtually pain-free, but at home he was liable to severe spasms if he simply stood up awkwardly from his lounge chair. When he relaxes, allowing the muscle tone of his torso to decrease, he becomes more likely to hurt himself in basic movements.

Lex has strong global muscles, so strong that they are covering a creeping weakness, and here's one clue: on the rare occasion Lex tries to sit directly on the ground, he grunts, moves awkwardly, and bumps down heavily. Those large muscles that should allow him to bend, twist, and fold have been otherwise employed in long-term bracing, co-contracting and fighting against gravity. Losing flexibility is an external sign of a more problematic issue. When Lex's global muscles decrease their activity, his local muscles do not protect his joints adequately, and then the pain starts.

If you can't bend, turn, or roll easily, you may well be employing global muscles in ongoing support to the detriment of your local muscles. If you have any muscles that feel like iron rods while you are simply standing, then you could be getting a message that your local muscles are under-engaged.

There is an alternative source of strength that is being neglected.

The Strength of Pressure

Fluid pressure (in both gases and liquids) is powerful. Think of the air pressure in tires that can support massive vehicles moving at great speed and hauling large weights, or the little hydraulic pumps that lift the end of a car to change one of those tires.

Hydraulic systems increase internal pressure to counter external pressure. In humans the main chamber of fluids is the abdomen. We can increase intra-abdominal pressure by activating the diaphragm, while the girdling abdominal muscles maintain a firm cylindrical wall. For the most part we don't notice the ebb and flow of intra-abdominal pressure. It is a gentle undulation coordinated with the rhythm of our breathing. However, for stronger work, attention to how we use this pressure is important.

Try It Yourself 7-2:
Release global muscles from support

Sit again on the firm stool or bench where you can easily lean back without obstruction. Sit upright with one hand on your lower abdomen and one hand on your chest.

Push your belly out into the hand that cups your lower abdomen. Think of this ball of fluid that is your abdomen roundly pushing into your hand, the bowl of your pelvis, and even back into your lumbar spine. The idea is to slightly expand the whole ball of the abdomen in every direction, not just toward your hand. Now tilt back, keeping your belly expanded. Use the hand on your chest to ensure that you do not sink your chest to keep your belly firm.

Notice how different it is to breathe with this way of tilting backward. What is your sense of effort or range as you tilt backward and return, while your abdomen is pushed consciously outward?

Try the first way again—simply tilting back without expanding the ball of your belly. Notice that as the abdominal muscles engage this way, they tend to compress the space between your hand and your spine, and it becomes more difficult to twist, turn, or side fold. As you repeat this, release one hand and raise that arm above your head—notice the weight of the arm as you lift.

Again push your belly into your hand as you tilt back, and see if it is easier to twist, turn, or fold as you continue to breathe in this movement. Again lift your arm above your head, and check if the experience of the weight is lighter or heavier.

If you can raise your arm lightly, your global muscles are available to take action that changes your shape easily. If your arm is heavy, you are still using global muscles for stability rather than action.

Compressing the Fluids, Not the Structure

We have described the cylinder of the torso in some detail; its width, length, and flexibility are important.

When we use intra-abdominal pressure well, the torso remains long, wide, deep, and adaptable. In the previous TIY you were asked to play with the idea of a round ball of fluid. Leaning back while maintaining a sense of the rounded ball pushing evenly into your hand, sides, and back allows twisting, turning, and folding to remain easy because your global muscles are still free to change your shape. Whereas if you draw your abdomen toward your spine as you lean back, you contract your major flexor and extensor groups simultaneously, causing several things to happen: your sense of length, width, and depth in the torso reduces, so your breath either halts or is labored, and flexibility diminishes. In this latter way of moving, both your fluids and your skeletal structure have been compressed.

OP2 and OP7 are inextricably linked: without good practice of skeletal alignment, the efficient use of intra-abdominal pressure becomes impossible (and vice versa). Fluids require space in three dimensions. Maintaining a sense of all three dimensions in space as you move is a way to reclaim power and reduce effort.

Lex's path to recovery was in relearning the dynamics of his torso, not by strengthening muscle groups—he was already strong—but looking for a response to pressure that expanded rather than compressed space—the experience of getting a bit taller and wider under load.

Grace A, at the beginning of OP2, had a similar issue. We mentioned that her abdominal muscles were chronically contracting. This constant engagement of flexors gradually brought her head and shoulders forward and down, in a computer-oriented hunch. These are visual signals, but equally concerning is the less visible disruption to fluid circulation through the torso—breath and motility are both limited by constant compression through the torso.

Pressure and Anxiety

"Clenching!" observed Rakel in her rehab session. She was being trained to notice the signals from her own system. It was a deceptively simple exercise—picking up objects of various weights. Six months earlier Rakel had fallen badly in a skiing accident. Ever since, she had experienced severe back pain that interfered with even the most routine chores of life. Now she was in a program to retrain her attention to physical signals. The most effective key she was finding was the sensation of her midsection contracting inward—or clenching.

The midsection is the area of our torso from the lower rim of the rib cage to a few centimeters below the belly button. When Rakel prepared to push or pull something heavy, she noticed this drawing inward was part of how she braced herself. Watching a suspenseful movie made her clench, driving her car next to a large truck on the freeway could elicit a similar response, as could disagreements at work. She was noticing just how many situations made her anxious, by observing when her breathing became shallow, her belly hardened, or she could feel her neck tightening. In fact there were so many parts of this clenching pattern that she wondered why she had never noticed it before.

Recognition was the first step. Now as soon as she called "clenching" she was being asked to stop and imagine her abdomen was a fluid-filled balloon. If she could activate her diaphragm so it slowly pushed down, flattening the top of the balloon, she would feel the pressure push out evenly into her back, front, sides, and down into the pelvis. When she did this, she could pick up heavy objects with no pain at all, her breathing would stay easy and her neck long. If she regressed to her clenching pattern, her tummy would suck inward, and her lower back would hurt.

Rakel had found that the mere thought of something that seemed too much could make her pull her belly in and sink her chest. For most people the anxiety response is "gut-clenching"—freezing the diaphragm and creating a shallow breathing pattern that saps ability.

Bea, the singer in the opening story of this chapter, also had an anxiety pattern. When she anticipated singing high notes she tightened through her belly, chest, and neck, virtually strangling her breath and sound. The trick of lifting the table required her to stabilize and organize her torso in a way that circumvented the constrictions. She could not deploy her habitual pattern while she was concurrently lifting. By the end of the workshop she had become aware that anxiety about her upper vocal range was sabotaging her physically.

Rakel and Bea worked with external weights (loads) to gradually relearn their responses to physical, mental, and emotional pressure. You might like to revisit TIY 4-1: Sense How Effort Spreads (p. 72), which demonstrated that effort was more likely to spread and immobilize regions when clenching a fist than when gripping and taking action with a hammer—even though the initial work in the fist was the same.

The Pressure of Contact

When a four-footed mammal is born, its mother will lick it all over: from top to tail and every square centimeter in between. This is not about hygiene; it's about stimulating the connections to the central nervous system through the skin. Human babies are not licked, but we are touched continuously, and from that moment forward the receptors in our skin and flesh begin a data flow to our central nervous system that does not cease until death. The tragic failure of orphanages in the nineteenth and twentieth centuries to provide nurturing touch resulted in horrendous mortality rates and demonstrated that caring tactile contact is essential for infant survival.

Tactile contact speaks directly to the nervous system. Exteroceptors from head to foot provide information on pressure, texture, temperature, and movement. As this principle is about the organizational importance of pressure, we will focus on that element.

We learn from a very young age to respond to differing pressures. With some attention to these responses we can begin to use the information to our advantage.

Try It Yourself 7-3:
Explore distal pressure and proximal organization

Sit on a comfortable chair, at a good height for standing and sitting.

Gently place your fingertips together—enough to feel the skin but not enough to depress the tip. Maintaining this delicate level of contact and sensitivity between your fingertips, raise one foot off the ground, then place it back down. Notice what you need to do as preparation to lift your leg a little while the fingers are joined in this way. Preparation might involve repositioning your feet, pelvis, torso, or head. As you lift the foot, notice the weight, any sensation of effort, and speed of the action, while you maintain the most delicate touch of the fingertips. Does your breathing remain free through the whole process, or did you find you needed to use some of the intra-abdominal pressure we have just discussed? Repeat a few times so you can gather as much information as possible about lifting your foot with the constraint of your fingertips lightly touching.

Now bring your palms together. Start with the palms touching as lightly as the fingertips so you can feel the skin-to-skin contact, then press a little more firmly so you are more aware of the flesh beneath the skin. There is a springiness to flesh that you can feel as you quietly pulse your palms together with a medium pressure. Do you feel anything changing in your intra-abdominal pressure as you hold your hands this way? Maintain this pressure as you again lift a foot. Do you need to prepare yourself in the same way as you did with the light touch? Are the weight, effort, and speed of your actions the same? Does your breathing remain unchanged through the entire action? Again repeat enough times to gather information about the whole process.

Finally, interlace your hands firmly so you can feel the bones of adjacent fingers. Your fingers can fold over the bony knuckles of the clasped hands. Again feel if there is any change to your torso when you do this—can you feel the possibility of your torso getting taller as you clasp your hands this way? Maintain this bony contact as you lift one foot. Once again pay attention to preparatory movements—do you need less or more? Do the weight, sensation of effort, and speed of your action increase or decrease? Is your breath freer or unchanged?

Of the three variations, which one allows your foot to lift most easily? Which way is lightest, fastest, and highest?

To touch lightly is a sophisticated level of any movement. If you have watched young children around animals, you will appreciate the many iterations required to learn light touch and gentle strokes. To contact with delicacy, where we can make distinctions about the texture and pressure of whatever we touch, requires us to have a solid base of support and a pelvic region organized for stability. For most people, lifting the foot while the hands are delicately touching is initially a movement conundrum. Considerable shifting of weight over the base goes on so that the foot/leg becomes light enough to lift from the floor. If you are involved in a pastime or job that requires light touch and delicate manipulation, consideration to stability at your feet and pelvic region—or even external ways to increase your base of support—is a great idea. This was touched on briefly in OP6, under "Using Tools" (p. 130).

At the other end of the spectrum is the firm touch we can have with hard surfaces. We used "skeletal" touch in the TIY, but you could equally use a coffee mug or bottle in hand to find that this type of pressure calls our system to a completely different organization, whereby our limbs become light and easy to lift with very little preparation. We can move our whole body with relative ease when our distal parts are sending a message of firm contact.

For those who would like to sense this idea more thoroughly, the entire TIY can be duplicated. Instead of using the contact between your hands, choose objects like a very delicate feathery or silky object for light touch, a malleable object that deforms with anything more than medium pressure, and a solid object like a coffee mug. Hold these as you go from sitting to standing instead of lifting a foot. See how the information of this touch organizes you to move.

Using Touch for Different Outcomes

A light touch is soothing. Instinctively humans use a soft and delicate stroking touch to soothe another's nervous system. To de-stress our own systems we can similarly use the stroking touch. Cat owners attest to the calming effect of stroking their cats after stressful days.

The simple action of feeling the texture of fur as you gently stroke along the coat lowers the tone of the arm, which generalizes eventually to the whole body. Others find a similar effect from feeling lush carpet with their bare feet. Lowering the tone of the hands and feet enough that we can perceive soft fibers, fur, delicate petals, or air or water passing fingers or toes gradually induces quieting of the whole system. In overwrought, overstressed, or generally busy lives it can be our quickest access to a timely respite.

Medium pressure—the sort you might use to handle a bunch of grapes, or to get your hands around a juicy hamburger without squirting contents in all directions—is wonderful for gathering information, for curiosity, and for exploration. You can still notice surface textures with this touch, but you are better set up to manipulate an object or feel beneath the surface to the shape and tone of muscles.

Firm contact prepares us for action. As we grasp unyielding surfaces our muscle tension increases, and local muscles firm up around joints to transmit force without shearing. It is literally bone deep. We become alert and more vigilant. It is this firmness of touch that is most likely to increase our intra-abdominal pressure, making us ready to shrink our base of support and move quickly.

Lex knows about firm pressure from his construction work—handling drills, hammer guns, and heavy loads keeps his grasp very strong. At the other end, his pets—a small aviary of birds—have taught him the importance of light touch. To hold a frightened small bird without damaging it, those work-hardened hands must be capable of a very delicate caress. But the middle ground is not quite as clear or practiced for him. His life has tended toward polarization between "on" and "off." His wife commented that he was either "flat out" or "out flat"—either at work or on the sofa.

Many people experience this issue with polarities, in all aspects of their lives. Yet our systems thrive on range. Lex was missing the middle range, which is where we learn to adapt, and he experienced pain when he tried to transition rapidly from "off" to "on." Just as our muscles and bones grow and strengthen in the "just right" zone of stress, so does the rest of us. This median area, where we can find ways to deal with pressure with neither underwhelm nor overwhelm, is important for our emotional, physical, and intellectual well-being. Concentrating on the quality of his transitions through the middle territories is an important part of Lex's recovery from pain.

LEARNING FROM THE INSIDE OUT

IN THE "LEARNING IN Focus" section of "Starting Points," we said that learning is wound implicitly through the seven organizing principles; learning and movement are entwined like the double helix of DNA. It's time now to be explicit about this relationship.

Our potential to direct our own lives—to fulfill our own intentions—is founded on the strength of these entwined strands.

It has long been understood that doing is a vital part of learning. A well-known Chinese axiom states: "I hear and I forget; I see and I remember; I do and I understand." Reflecting this axiom, and as a counter to Western emphasis on academic learning, "Just do it" has become an important slogan. It's a good start, but to really understand,

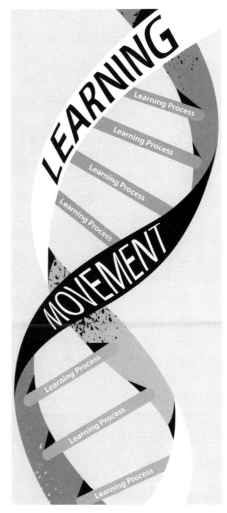

FIGURE 56: A model of learning and movement

to decrease frustration and accelerate ability, *how* we do it is paramount.
If we can understand how processes of learning interlock with our ways
of doing, we can literally do what we set our minds and actions to. That's
why, in our model, learning processes are the two-way threads that bond
learning and movement.

The Power of Processes

Ari is doing well at university now, but for several years this seemed
unlikely to ever happen. He had been in a downward spiral in
high school, becoming more and more sullen with each grade. He
hated math especially. His father, who had never struggled academ-
ically, was at a loss. Desperate to stop the slide, he found a tutor,
Seth, who was reputed to be very gifted in math, though somewhat
unconventional.

To his father's puzzlement, Ari spent the next four months
playing soccer with Seth. Ari started smiling again, and his soccer
improved markedly. He became a more versatile and strategic player,
but this didn't change his math scores. His father remained concerned. Then one day, early in the fifth month, Ari asked Seth to
help him with a math problem. For the rest of the year the tutorials
ranged across the different academic subjects, with a little soccer
thrown in regularly. By the end of the year Ari not only had an A in
math, he had improved in all his subjects beyond the expectation of
his teachers.

Delighted but still puzzled, Ari's father asked Seth why he'd spent
so long on soccer and not math in the early months. The tutor smiled.
"We were following Ari's curiosity. He liked soccer, so we worked
with aspects of his own skills and then together we'd analyze parts of
his teammates' and opponents' games. As soon as Ari asked if some of
the ideas might be useful for learning other things, we could open the
books." Ari's questions set the timing.

Curiosity is a powerful intrinsic motivator for learning. We
can all learn without curiosity—this is many people's experience
of formal education. But the struggle we experience when lacking

intrinsic motivation can gradually transform into resistance to schooling, education, and even the idea of learning. It may seem counterintuitive, but for Ari the long detour via soccer became the scenic shortcut to academic success.

Josh Waitzkin, in *The Art of Learning*, provides another perspective on this. Josh discovered chess in a public park at the age of six. Thereafter he played and practiced chess with such fervor that he achieved the title of International Master at the age of sixteen. A movie was made of his *wunderkind* rise, but the fame and expectations that followed eroded his passion for the cerebral world of chess tournaments. In his early twenties, curiosity took him into a martial arts class as a raw beginner. In less than a decade he was again winning world titles, this time for tai chi. He found transferability not in the subject matter but in the learning processes he used for practice and mastery.

Seven Learning Processes

With help, both Ari and Josh found deeper structures in one subject that could transfer across physical and intellectual disciplines: they discovered processes. Many people focus only on subject matter, on form and details, never quite noticing that how they learn is separate from what is being learned.

Processes are the "how": ways, methods, or strategies that can be applied to many arenas. For instance, the scientific method is a set of processes (hypothesize, test, observe, and review) for conducting research. The method describes how to research, without restricting what is researched, which of course ranges from microbiology to musicology and beyond. Similarly entrepreneurs use processes—business strategies—to build businesses in widely different sectors and activities.

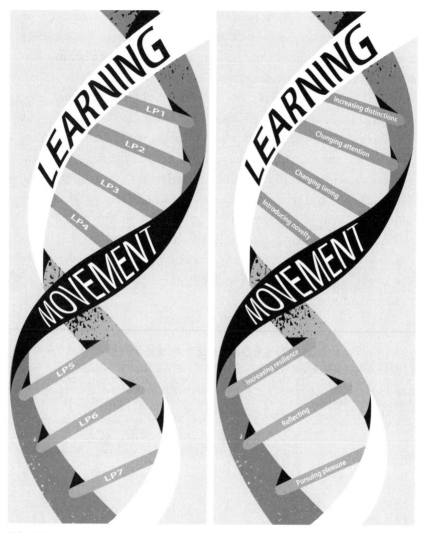

FIGURE 57: A model of learning, learning processes, and movement

Ari spent four months apparently just playing soccer with his tutor. Seth's unconventional approach was to build Ari's awareness of how he was learning in the one area he loved—his soccer. To use something consciously you must first become aware of it. Over time, Ari had a glimmer that learning itself may be transferable—the observations, analysis, and trials he was using for improving his soccer might be applied to different subjects—even to studying math.

Learning processes (LPs) are neither subject- nor discipline-specific. They are always transferable. As Josh showed, skills as different as chess and tai chi can be mastered using the same learning processes. Eminent educator Guy Claxton, in *Wise Up: The Challenge of Lifelong Learning*, summarizes getting better at learning as "getting better at knowing when, how, and what to do when you don't know what to do.[1] This is the purpose of processes. We outline here the seven most valuable processes for sensory learning.

LP1: Increasing Distinctions

In "Starting Points" we discussed the power of distinctions to separate ideas by defining differences and to unify ideas by finding common ground. In OP4 we explained that distinctions "are the rich data a learning nervous system feasts on." Both perspectives begin with the ability to discriminate.

A gulf between novice and expert in any field is the ability first to sense keener distinctions and then to use that information: the champion archer who discerns and adjusts for changes in wind and barometric pressure; the musician who manipulates small shifts in timbre, rhythm, and pace to create subtle interpretive inflections; or the woodworker who carves a single, long, sweeping arc, continuously adjusting for the changing grain and resistance of the wood, without lifting the chisel from the groove.

Very often the novice will not even know there is a distinction to be made. We must recognize that these differences exist before we can learn the subtle sensations of barometric pressure, vibration of timbre, or resistance from wood grain. Throughout the TIYs in this book we have asked you to notice differences that may at first have escaped your attention. Most recently, in TIY 7-3: Explore Distal Pressure and Proximal Organization (p. 142), we asked you to discern a subtle difference in how you stood

---

[1] Claxton develops the concept of "learning power" in a number of works. *Wise Up* makes an excellent starting point.

up, depending on the contact between your hands. You need many of the following learning processes for that distinction to become clear and easily discernible in multiple situations, but the starting point is knowing that such a distinction exists, and that you can search your sensations for it.

Making clearer distinctions about emotions—our feelings—may be the most potent area for practicing discernment. How we feel about something will make all the difference to our approach and capacity. Ari hated math, but at the end of four months, something had changed in his feelings and he could begin to think about math with curiosity. In her excellent book *How Emotions Are Made*, Lisa Feldman Barrett speaks of making fine distinctions as "increasing granularity," referencing photography where finer grain (more pixels) creates a clearer picture. She explores the science behind the surprising research findings that people who have more words for distinctions between emotions have consistently better academic, social, and health outcomes.

At the end of many TIYs we included an instruction to notice how you felt after following the sequence. This is a moment to take stock of sensations and emotions, and to experience differences that may escape your daily attention. Expanding the scope and number of distinctions you make in your sensations, feelings, thoughts, and actions has far-reaching consequences.

Feedback in Focus

A distinction on its own can feel like a "so what" experience. To release its power, we need feedback.

An archer receives direct external feedback when the arrow hits or misses the target. But before releasing the arrow, the experienced archer has made multiple adjustments based on internal feedback: their standing balance, the "just right" grip to draw the bow, aligning the torso to achieve the desired trajectory, and so on. Our nervous systems are always tracking the variances between what is wanted/needed and what is happening. Not only do we use the immediate sensations from external and internal sources, but we compare with prior experiences and perceived ideals. We are predicting, comparing, and adjusting continuously, and mostly below the threshold of our conscious awareness.

This "predict, act, compare, and adjust" feedback loop exists at every level of our systems, for both voluntary and involuntary functions. The latter are our life-supporting systems, which are self-balancing (homeostatic) and operate below conscious direction. Between these and our voluntary actions, like walking and running, there lies a much wider range of movements where we can sense and amplify feedback more than most of us have ever dreamt. In an extraordinarily moving piece, Dr. Norman Doidge relates the story of Cheryl, whose vestibular system was irreparably damaged, so she felt like she was perpetually falling. For years her system had been continuously searching and failing to find confirmation that she was upright and stable, so she staggered like a drunk even when holding a wall. Through an ingenious process she learned to balance using sensory feedback from her tongue.[2]

Expanding discernment of the gray zone between voluntary and involuntary function is a rich reservoir. In Stef's story about overcoming plantar fasciitis (OP5) she had to learn to perceive a great many distinctions that had at first been invisible to her conscious sensing. Through constant experimentation and feedback, she discovered how the movement of the pelvis and spine was implicated in the plantar fasciitis:

> *When Stef slowed down her walk, she could begin to feel how, in parts of the transfer, her pelvis and lower spine stiffened, which caused her foot to "grasp" at the ground. It was subtle, but as she trained her attention on the initiation of each step, she was able to detect the difference between gliding the pelvis forward in continuous motion and inhibiting some of the pelvic mobility.*

A vital part of the feedback loop is our environment. Stef's subtle exploration of sensation in her spine and pelvis used the contact of her

---

[2] This précis does no justice to the story, so if this area of neuroplasticity intrigues you, please read Doidge's book.

foot with the ground as crucial information. There is continual feedback from our environment, not all of which is physical—or helpful or healthful. Many of us learned early to tie particular sensory information to emotional interpretations. These interpretations may trigger a craving for, or aversion to, the stimulus. In this way, the glance of a stranger, the judgments of an "authority," or the compliments of a friend can send us into unwarranted emotional spirals, changing every other aspect of our movement.

As we recognize and distinguish between increasingly subtle internal and external stimuli, more choices of response are available. Feedback helps us sort, choose, and use. We can process information from the present moment, access sensory-rich memories, and combine these to predict near or distant futures, generalize current situations, or imagine alternative scenarios.

Repetition and Variety

"Gently repeat," "try this several times," "return again"—these are all exhortations that recur constantly through the TIYs. Repetition is essential for learning. Another way of saying this is the oft-repeated mantra of neuroplasticity: "neurons that fire together wire together."

However, doing the same thing the same way many times is highly inefficient for learning. Building variation into exercises not only helps us stay attentive and aware but also increases the comparison points for making better distinctions. This is why you will see instructions like the following from TIY 6-2: Let Your Foot Direct Your Torso (p. 126).

Keep repeating this small 5–10 percent of the movement. Each time you repeat you can make it simpler and lighter.

In OP4 we spoke about gym-loving Riya and her search for stamina. She had a varied regime but was not using distinctions or variation within each choice, particularly in weight training. After her friend mentioned her audible breathing, Riya began to vary how she initiated lifting to discover the source of the altered breathing and tension. The results of the process were so outstanding she continued it:

> *Riya continues her investigation of decreasing effort at the gym. For most people this would be a strange place to practice effortlessness; however, it is a fabulous playground for experimenting with spreading load, using less force to achieve better results. She can take sneak peeks at how others work and compare how they coordinate themselves to achieve an exercise with how she is doing it.*

Repetition with variety accelerates learning. Each exercise session is an opportunity to be curious, to experiment like a scientist, to hypothesize, test, observe, and review. Small changes in initiation, speed, direction, or weight placement, when matched with curiosity about the difference they make, can yield big results. It is more important to feel differences within the variations than to be able to describe them. We can notice and learn something long before we can label it.

There are many ways to build variation into whatever you are doing. This keeps your thinking engaged in the sensory motor domain rather than busy in abstraction. Variety is not just the spice of life, it is sustenance for our nervous systems.

LP2: Changing Attention

The ability to make distinctions is reliant on attention. So here we must make an important distinction. Soldiers are drilled in "coming to attention" and children commanded at school to "pay attention." In both cases, attention is accompanied by a stiff, constrained posture and eyes fixed on an external source. This externally commanded attention is very different from the self-directed attention for learning we spoke of in "Starting Points": "that moment when we bring our sensors (internal and/or external) to focus on a point of interest." It is the external we will focus on here.

There are two main aspects we will consider: first what we pay attention to, and second how we move our attention.

Our sensory systems are streaming more information through our nervous system than we can possibly attend to at any moment. Little wonder that, without training, attention is guided largely by habit and circumstance and only minimally by choice.

We all have habitually dominant sensory sources. For some it's the internal world—the interoceptors, vestibular, or proprioceptors—while others are more attuned to the external world through the teleceptors and/or exteroceptors, as we explained in OP1. Within each group is a narrower range that we habitually attend to, shaped by our history and interests. For example, a gymnast may consistently search for distinctions in the angle of joints (proprioception) but have very little awareness of breathing (interoception).

Understanding your personal habits of attention, and how they are modified by tasks and environment, can yield surprising information. In OP4 we discussed Dianne's experience of changing her modes of attention. Brought up on external visual and verbal feedback, she needed time and practice to expand her range of attention:

She had never developed her attention to the internal experience of movement, in fact she had consciously suppressed it, to reduce the unpleasant aspects of long hours in training. Experiencing her actions as sensations and breaking the reliance on mirrors took a long time. It was both uncomfortable and liberating. At first she was full of doubt, but she learned to listen to internal information with growing confidence. As her trust in her own senses grew, the uncertainty and fragility she had thought were normal diminished.

Just as tasks and environments influence what we attend to, they also impact how we move our attention. Imagine for a moment a busy restaurant kitchen at peak time. There are many activities to be seen, aromas to be smelled, and noises to be heard from many directions. The amount and type of sensory information you notice would differ according to your role. If you were the head chef, a hygiene inspector, or a dishwasher on your first day, your attention would be drawn to very different things. Your success and safety would depend on how rapidly you could gather diverse but relevant information.

Such a hectic environment would activate your externally oriented sensors but would leave little room for interoception or reflection. If you return home after a busy working day to discover escalating aches and pains, it could be because the signals from your body, suppressed by constant external focus during the day, can now be perceived.

Relieved of time stress and saturated sensors we might begin to practice moving attention to expand awareness.

Try It Yourself: Sense yourself

Stand comfortably—what do you attend to? What do you make distinctions about?

Teleceptors. What do you see, hear, smell around you? Is one of these senses more finely tuned than the others? Look around you and notice the shadows that lie next to every object, giving rise to your perception of depth and dimension. Search for aromas near you, noticing the change in how your head moves when led by your nose scanning for scent. Now tune into sounds—close and far, loud or soft—and again notice how your head orients in a subtly different way. Imagine yourself standing in the kitchen of a busy restaurant at peak time. Reflecting on your habits, which of your teleceptors would you pay more attention to?

Exteroceptors. How do you feel your contact with the ground through your feet? How is the pressure distributed over different parts of your feet, and how much of your foot is interacting with the ground as you make the minute changes necessary to keep balanced? Are there differences between your left and right sides? Can you feel the different textures and pressures of fabric against your skin? What about the different temperatures of your skin as you stand, some parts of your body covered and others open to the air? Imagine you are standing on the deck of a boat. How would different types of weather influence your awareness of your feet on the deck, or the direction of the wind on your skin, as your balance is challenged by the motion?

Interoceptors. How do you sense the movement of your breathing? What movements are you tracking when you sense rhythm, timing, or ease of breathing? How would you sense your breathing if you imagined someone was watching you? If you started skipping on the spot where you stand, what parts of your breathing might come to your awareness when skipping fast or slow? What internal sensations might you sense once you had stopped?

Proprioceptors. How do you sense the arrangement of your limbs, head, and torso—their length and width, their sense of "stacking up" to support you in standing? Imagine the lines of your four limbs and the line of your spine and head—that's five lines. If you reached your right hand toward your left knee, how would you track the changing arrangement of these five lines? As the lines curve and reorient, are some parts of you clearer in your image? Would it become difficult to track parts of yourself when doing something more challenging, like a somersault?

Vestibular system. Where is your head in space? Where does it orient? Is there any tilting—slightly up/down, left/right? How easy it is it to move your head through the cardinal directions—forward/back, up/down, and left/right? If you think about a difficult task, perhaps the somersault again, how mobile is your head? If you feel unsafe or unbalanced, what happens to your head and its ability to move?

What is your general sense of standing and walking now, after bringing your attention to more sensory information? Has it changed something in your image of yourself and what can be included as you move? Would it influence your awareness of the environment or your actions within the environment?

Different senses are called forward at different times, but did this TIY demonstrate any habitually accessed sensors? Any virtual blind spots? Attending to more sensory sources increases distinctions and feedback to our nervous system, which increases possible responses and options. "Stop and smell the roses" is not just sage advice to slow down and appreciate the moments of your life, but to practice attention to your environment and yourself.

We can simultaneously distinguish features of our internal state and external environment. Expanding the range of our attention is training for a more global state of awareness, from which we can appreciate multiple perspectives and make more conscious choices.

Foreground, Background, and Pain

Learning to direct your own attention is at the heart of millennia-old meditation practices and current mindfulness techniques. Its practice, backed by compelling research, now has a significant role in pain management.

Intense pain demands attention. It takes over the foreground of our thoughts, emotions, and sensations. This is necessary in acute situations, but when pain persists into a chronic state this focus is debilitating.

We have established that we habitually attune to only a narrow band of the information available to our sensory systems. When chronic pain dominates this band, life becomes a grinding endurance test. Widening and moving attention does not deny or suppress pain but diminishes its dominance.

We can think of sensory layers as foreground and background. Just as in a photograph, where subjects in the foreground are bigger, brighter, and clearer than background details, so too is pain magnified when it has hijacked our foreground. The quality of a sensation changes when it is relegated to the background. Visually objects diminish in relative size, vibrancy, and clarity as they recede; so too sensations, including pain, diminish in urgency as the spotlight of our attention moves away.

When focusing on single sensations, we can observe detail and make distinctions. As we include more sensations, diminishing the central focus, we find relationships and perspective. The key skill is shifting your attention.

In OP6 we spoke about Lao, who was experiencing debilitating pain when he returned to driving his taxi after having broken his ribs. His grandmother used direct touch to change the location of his attention.

This change not only diminished the pain, it also expanded his range of movement and triggered an ongoing engagement with his own recovery:

> *For the next few minutes she placed her sharp fingers at different points of Lao's spine and made him turn his head from that point. Then she did the same to get him bowing his head forward and back and to either side. "Move your head like juggling a plate on a long bamboo stick—from here!" One last time she prodded his tailbone. Lao had the message, loud and clear. His next driving shift changed from an endurance test to an adventure in how many opportunities he could find to turn and tilt his head from different parts of himself, right down to his ankles.*

For us to move without pain or restriction, the curves of our spine need to adjust continuously to the demands of our actions. Unfortunately the trauma of injury and the process of recovery can overwrite our original healthy but unconscious patterns of movement, leaving us stuck in discomfort and effort. Attention is a tool to lead us back consciously from the sticking point to ease.

We all get stuck—not just in our patterns of moving but in our habits of thinking and even in our range of emotions. Like any other skill, attention is an ability we can improve. Finding ways to explore more aspects of your movement and your environment, lightly, with curiosity, and without judgment, releases us from many painful fixations and opens new possibilities.

When our attention expands into awareness, we feel calm but engaged. It is not a state we can live in constantly, but it is a state all self-directed learners cultivate.

LP3: Changing Timing

There is no aspect of how we live, move, or learn that is not touched by time—time as a span, time as a pace, and time as a sequence are particularly pertinent to learning.

It takes time to learn. While learning a set of facts may take very little time, to learn how those facts can be applied in different ways takes a longer time span. A child introduced to a ball may quickly learn to kick, but kicking with power and precision takes a long time, and learning to "bend it like Beckham"[3] takes even longer.

When we give ourselves time, we can attain a depth and breadth of understanding that were inconceivable in the first flush of learning. Again there is an axiom that covers this concept: "We overestimate what can be achieved in one year and underestimate what can be achieved in ten."[4] This suggests the compounding nature of learning over time. Yet our society doles out labels such as "stupid," "slow," "incapable," and "lacking aptitude" to anyone who doesn't grasp a subject within an arbitrarily selected timeframe. These undeserved labels can last for life, sabotaging further attempts to self-direct learning.

Speed and rhythm give us a different perspective on timing. We each have our own pace for different functions—from breathing to walking to brushing our teeth. We also have favored paces for learning. "Slow" is perhaps the most undervalued and least respected pace in our present society, but it is extremely important neurologically for the development of awareness.

Stef, whose story we told in OP5 and mentioned earlier, had to slow down significantly to discern the subtle stiffening of spine and pelvis when she stepped forward. This was pivotal in her learning about the plantar fasciitis. When there are many distinctions to be made, or significant internal attention required, we need to slow our pace. The prefrontal cortex, the part of the brain processing this type of information, is slower relative to other regions.

The ultimate slowdown is a pause. Not only is our prefrontal cortex slow, but it is energy-hungry. It needs intervals to virtually "wipe the slate clean," rest, and reset. Like a palate cleanser between courses or a break between paragraphs, we need gaps to signal something has

---

[3] This is the title of and a line from a popular 2002 British movie referring to a kick that produces an unexpectedly curved trajectory of the ball, a signature move of British soccer player David Beckham.

[4] This phrase, used in business and personal-development workshops, is often attributed to Bill Gates, founder of Microsoft, but we have been unable to find an accurate citation.

finished and something new will begin. In TIY 5-3: Imagine Your
Spine (p. 97), you were using mental imagery along with attention to
interoception, so we were very specific about using the pause:

> *Pause for a moment, just to walk without an image in mind before you
> try the next one.*

Pausing can be a full stop, a total rest, or it can be using a neutral
activity, like walking, without a particular intention or attention.

All activities can be paused, but not all activities can be slowed
down. Chopping wood, for instance, requires momentum. You can
learn an axe-swing slowly and refine the action with attentive repetition, but chopping with enough force to cut wood requires a level of
power and momentum that you can't practice slowly.

Fast rhythms also have a place in the learning repertoire. "Fast"
requires us to break up patterns of conscious control, habits of tension,
hyperfocus, or even timidity. To go really fast we must stop trying,
stop thinking, and just do, which is an illuminating experience for
anyone who achieves it.

When you are getting frustrated in learning, whatever the subject
matter, it is always worth trying a change of pace to see what difference this can make.

Last there is time as a flow: the sequence of learning. In Ari's case,
his tutor introduced math only when Ari demonstrated enough curiosity to ask a question about using his soccer strategies for learning
math. This is an aspect of time that excellence in teaching and learning can pivot on. "Don't run before you can walk" and "A stitch in
time saves nine" are proverbs about time as sequence at its most basic.
For example, taking time to learn good form before speeding up or
adding power to movement can prevent many injuries and accelerate
skills acquisition—though that seems paradoxical to many novices.
The more sophisticated use of sequence demonstrated by Ari's tutor,
Seth, requires greater knowledge of yourself or the individual you are
working with. Introduce a challenge too soon and the learner can be
overwhelmed, too late and they may have "turned off," dismissing fertile territory as irrelevant.

LP4: Introducing Novelty

Novelty is one of the conditions for triggering neuroplastic change mentioned in "Starting Points" under "Neuroplasticity." The best teachers, trainers, and coaches use novelty to engage or re-engage the attention of students or trainees. It is no mere trick to entertain but a call to alertness for the nervous system. It is the flint for sparking curiosity and preparing the brain for new connections.

We began OP7 with the story of Bea, a singer who was having difficulty with high notes. She expected vocal exercises; instead she was asked first to lift a table, then to lift it while singing. Not only did the results startle her, but the novelty of the approach caused her to reassess what she knew and had tried previously:

> *Bea and the onlookers were astounded: her voice sailed strongly through the whole passage, steady, clear, and true. Somehow the lifting task had organized her breathing and singing in a way no focus on parts or mechanisms had ever done.*

The workshop leader had a systemic view of singing, broader than others Bea had encountered. But of course not all novelty is about changing paradigms. Novelty is by definition something new, but newness can be encountered in many ways—changing one element or changing position can be enough to create a novel experience.

Constraining an Element

Very simply, constraining one element of a habitual action can encourage us to discover more options, challenging the brain to find another pathway. For generations "lazy eye" (amblyopia) in children has been treated using a constraint: the stronger (dominant) eye is covered with a patch to coerce the child's system into coordinating sight with the weaker eye.

TIY 4-6: Find Clues in the Non-habitual (p. 85) asked you to cut paper with one constraint: using your nondominant hand. As you practiced cutting this way, you were asked to notice all the odd, extraneous movements that can accompany our first attempts at coordination. The constraint returns you to being a novice, and if we do this with the attention and discernment of proficient learners, many things can be discovered.

. . . notice what the experience of cutting with this side feels like. So much more than the hand is activated as you cut. Your whole arm is involved, as is the way you hold your neck and head, and where you shift your weight. Many people tighten their jaw and thereby inhibit breath. If you attend closely enough you may even find your attitude (thinking and feeling) is different when you cut with this side.

Changing Orientation

A significant issue in all forms of education is situational learning—what we learn in one environment does not necessarily transfer into another. For example, the knowledge diligently learned for exams often seems to evaporate in real life, until it is relearned and practiced anew.

In OP5 we spoke about Sue learning to drive at night. When riding a bicycle, she knew to keep her eyes on her path and not on the obstacles she wanted to avoid. Yet in the car, she had to relearn this before she could generalize it further.

This . . . jogged an old memory of learning to ride a bike. She had constantly ridden into poles and holes until she had learned to keep her eyes on the path she wanted to follow, and not on the obstacle she wanted to avoid. Now it appeared she had fallen into the old habit of looking where she didn't want to go—the oncoming traffic. She had to make a concerted effort to look at the very center of the lane ahead of her. Sue did get the hang of night driving and did get her license. She has continued to notice how often in life people are coached to keep their eye on the ball, or the target, or the finish line, or the prize.

We need to have experiences in multiple orientations/environments to generalize our abilities.

In TIY 1-1: Revisit Sucking and Swallowing (p. 20), though we didn't ask you to change your orientation, we finished with these comments:

Imagine how many times, and in how many positions, you practiced sucking as a baby—and how you became stronger and more efficient at it.

In time, and as you were fed in different positions, you learned to use
more coordinated movements of the whole body. The organization of
abdominal activity, breathing, and swallowing became sophisticated
enough to carry on these activities in many positions, diverse combina-
tions, and with varying intensity.

If you wish, you can return to TIY 1-1 and explore how lying on
your back, your side, or your front creates a different set of experiences. Novel orientations change your relationship to gravity, and
therefore different muscles must be activated at different intensi-
ties; they change your relationship to your environment, so sensors give different information. In our foundation fable of the seven
blind men and the elephant, each man experienced the elephant
from a different orientation, profoundly changing his image of the
elephant (the world). Each shift in orientation can potentially add
more information to your self-image by creating new possibilities
in your thinking, sensing, and—if repeated often enough—in your
neurology.

LP5: Increasing Resilience

Self-directed learning is no easy task. We need motivation, curiosity,
and some pleasurable rewards to keep going. How do we continue
after setbacks? How do we persevere when the time we are investing
or the many repetitions needed—even spiced up with variety—seem
too onerous in a world of distractions? Through these minor hur-
dles, and especially when major traumas have not just set us back but
knocked us far from our original course, we need resilience.

Recognizing and cultivating the thoughts, actions, and feelings that
help us keep going builds resilience. And when we can recognize the
conditions in which we are most receptive to new information, then we
can duplicate them at will.

Moving easily to satisfy curiosity or desire is a great state for
learning. Infants return to this state continuously in their journey to
an upright stance. We could say it is an ideal state, but we cannot
say it's essential. We learn in all manner of ways. For young and old,

frustration can be a tremendous provocation to learn. Ambition, competition, and compulsion are also powerful drivers. Fear, too, can be a learning state—but the lessons we embody are unpredictable.

Challenge vs. Threat

Challenge can be exciting: a little new, a little edgy, piquing our curiosity and sense of competition with ourselves or others. Or, at the other end of the scale, it can be a "fight or flight"–provoking challenge that seems to (or maybe does) threaten our lives. The difference between an invigorating challenge and a debilitating threat is very individual—dependent on our personal history and current abilities.

In OP1 we discussed Estelle, who as she slowly lost her sight gradually found her world a more and more threatening place:

> . . . *when she took hold of a guiding arm her whole body stiffened with fear of the unseen. She gripped with an almost clawed hand; she drew her arm firmly in to her side, and the muscles surrounding her rib cage contracted, as if ready to hunker down. This stiffening robbed her of responsiveness, making guiding difficult. The defensiveness she embodied physically also colored her social interactions, and she had gradually become reclusive.*

When she was re-introduced to an activity she had loved, where she could playfully embrace challenges, it created the time, safety, and motivation to soften and reconfigure her responses.

> *Muscles that were once held tight to stabilize are now free to respond. The threats to Estelle's safety haven't changed, but her ability to deal with them has.*

For most of us, somewhere along the spectrum between challenge and threat is a point where we can keep our faculties of attention and discernment, embrace the novel, and move with ease to trial and error. When Estelle found this in a theatre group, though the external conditions of her life didn't change, her perception of threat did—she became more resilient.

Embracing Incompetence

As we grow up, many of us experience increasing discomfort with appearing to be ignorant or incompetent. "I don't know" becomes a shameful admission rather than an invitation for discovery. Yet recognizing what we don't know is an imperative step in learning: it is the first great step in the learning cycle. We need emotional resilience to bear not knowing.

The "four stages of competence" is a simple model of a learning hierarchy.[5] The model proposes four major stages for mastery of a skill:

1. Unconscious incompetence (we don't know what we don't know). We need something or someone to draw our attention to our ignorance before we can move to . . .

2. Conscious incompetence (we know what we don't know). At this stage it becomes apparent what we need to learn so we can use all our processes to scope out and acquire new skills. We move toward . . .

3. Conscious competence (knowing what we know). We can practice our competence many times and in multiple ways until it "becomes second nature" and we reach . . .

4. Unconscious competence (we no longer notice our knowing). Our competence becomes so habitual it sinks from our consciousness.

This is a cyclic (or spiral) journey, so even as we enter stage four of a skill, we may begin again to butt up against the next level of unconscious incompetence.

Climbing the levels of skill and knowledge in any endeavor takes perseverance—the ability to weather the setbacks of our ineptitude or ignorance. With resilience we can accept our incompetence, knowing it is neither permanent nor defining; it is simply a step in the process of learning.

---

[5] The four stages of competence is variously attributed, so we have not cited a source.

At any time, we are all at different stages of competence with different skills. For those who suffer from "impostor syndrome" (thinking "I'm a fake/I'll be found out"), this can be a settling idea. While it may be hard to imagine for some people, feeling incompetent can become an exciting signal that you have found new territory for your curious self to explore.

LP6: Reflecting

In the "Neuroplasticity" section of "Starting Points" we wrote:

> *Neuroplasticity is a property of our brains that does not discriminate good from bad. We are all capable of repeating novel activities, with attention and with elevated emotions, that will have a negative impact on our lives. Our best chance for positive outcomes is to be aware of what we do, how we do it, and our clear intentions.*

Here's another way to put it: our best chance for positive outcomes is reflection—the essential step where we assess results and choose to discard or reinforce the direction we've taken.

Pausing is key. In the unrelenting grip of action, it is easy to disengage from the process of learning without noticing. A short pause allows an opportunity to recognize and reset both attitude and attention. A longer pause gives us time to reflect more broadly. And a rest of hours or days is important for integrating information at a deeper, systemic level.

In William's story, in OP3, we looked at a defining moment when reflecting had potentially shaped his career. William was the small boy who couldn't walk across a log like his classmates but resorted to scooting on his bottom.

> *. . . when he was finally across, he rose from the log feeling ashamed and unwilling to look anyone in the eye.*

> *. . . the greatest surprise from this event came at the end of the day when the group gathered round the campfire. William was singled out for bravery. . . . That he had been smart enough to find a way to keep moving, despite his fear, had earned him the respect of the organizers. According to William's recollection, that day has significantly informed his approach to teaching, and perhaps even his choice to teach.*

Had those initial reactions of burning shame not been challenged by additional information—the admiration of the organizers—and deepened by reflection over time, William believes his career direction would have been entirely different.

William's story represents the impact of reflection over long time spans. But the short spans are also important. We have seeded the TIYs of this book not just with suggestions for pausing, but with content for reflection. Like any other skill, reflection needs to be practiced repeatedly and with variety. Here are some "seeds" from TIY 3-1: Explore Spinal Movements (p. 52).

Pause. Take a moment of rest to notice your comfort level in this position now. Has the sensation of lying on the towel changed at all?

This is an encouragement to pause between actions, to experience the aftermath of action, and to compare "before and after" sensations.

Achieving these light undulations can take time. Return with curiosity at different times of day, or different parts of the week, until you feel the aesthetic pleasure of discovering a primal movement that began before birth.

A deeper form of reflection is simply to rest and reset: dispense with the thoughts and allow our genius nervous system to sort through the repercussions and refine, clarify, or create new connections. Moments, minutes, hours, or days later you can return afresh to the movements, scanning for change in ease or accessibility, or noticing confusion, gaps, or disruptions perhaps for the very first time.

Attention to differences of quality, efficiency, and satisfaction separates learning from exercise.

This last "seed" is an exhortation to be expansive with your reflections, ranging from the particular to the general. At the end of a TIY, when you have been engaged in a quiet, introspective sensory process—a very distinctive learning state—you may be well placed to engage in expansive, integrative reflection.

Ultimately transfer of learning takes place in the spaces between the actions, ideas, and feelings. It takes place in the time we give ourselves to reflect.

LP7: Pursuing Pleasure

Finally, the pursuit of pleasure for learning should not be underestimated. Pleasure is an important stimulant for our brain: it fires curiosity and motivation and generally makes tasks easier. We may learn in many conditions, and in many ways, but who wouldn't want to expand their repertoire for learning with pleasure?

We'll return once more to Ari and Seth, from the start of this chapter. Since soccer was what Ari loved, his tutor used this as the entry point to learning. Pursuing his pleasure in soccer, Ari was happy to consciously learn and improve. Once he had the skills to improve something he already enjoyed, he found the confidence to apply the new strategies to the school subjects he found difficult.

It's easy to recognize young children taking pleasure in learning. You will see them playfully involved with whatever has engrossed them: not overstimulated and seeking attention, not grimly compulsive, but quietly attentive to their own curiosities.

We can look back to that childlike state and find some pointers for ourselves. Every now and then you might practice playfulness where you have goals but can detach from when, how, or even if you achieve them. You could seek out a state of ease and reversibility, where you feel ready to try a challenge without compulsion. You can play with different physical, emotional, or psychological perspectives without attaching irrevocable meaning to them.

You could find your pleasure and allow that to set your guideposts for learning.

PRINCIPLES INTO PRACTICE

POPULAR WISDOM RECOGNIZES THAT tourists will explore more of a region in a few days than many of its citizens will explore in decades. Most of us similarly approach our bodies and our movement. We allow visitors (doctors, therapists, teachers, instructors, and coaches) to explore and be more expert about ourselves than we are. The principles in this book are designed for your own explorations, to pique your curiosity, highlight the "must-sees" and "must-dos" of yourself as a moving human. To become an expert on yourself, you need time exploring, revisiting, reading, and doing, seeking recommendations and trying them out.

We started this book with an explorer's story: we added a seventh blind man to the traditional fable of the blind men and the elephant—one who found a more active way of investigating the unfamiliar.

Our aim in adding the seventh blind man was never to make the six blind men wrong. There is strength and wisdom in learning one aspect in detail—in confining attention and specializing. Each man would have raised the wonder and appreciation of the crowd as he expounded his discoveries. Our principles too can be studied alone. Each reader will have favorites, understood more easily and applied more readily to your life or another's. Returning to your favorite until you recognize its many aspects is an excellent process.

The seventh man in our parable climbed the tree intending to reach the elephant from above. He meant to calmly explore the beast in much the same way as his fellow philosophers but from an alternative orientation. However, pandemonium arose with the arguing below and the seventh blind man rode the elephant, not by intention but by accident. His curiosity had taken him to a place where this became a possibility.

Each time we begin our explorations from a novel place, new possibilities can arise. The chances for discovery and integration increase.

Such explorations can also be a disaster. Our seventh man might have fallen or been thrown from the elephant. He might have stayed rigid and felt nothing more than the surging chemicals of emotion. Trying something different has never been for the faint-hearted. Safe exploring is at the heart of the principles of quality and learning.

Like the parts of an elephant, each principle may be recognizably different but also inseparably part of the whole. Good use of structure requires good balance. Dynamic balance emerges from successfully integrated developmental stages. We will never complete the developmental sequence if we cannot find the special relationship between the head and the pelvis, and so on. The principles do not operate in isolation.

Feldenkrais: A Framework for Learning

As mentioned in "Starting Points," this material was first presented as webinars for an audience of Feldenkrais practitioners. Though the principles do not belong to the Feldenkrais Method, our thinking and approach have been strongly influenced by the method. Following are some of the most salient aspects of the method and the man, which may help clarify our perspective.

Moshe Feldenkrais, the method's founder, had two definitions of health.

First, he held that health is the ability to recover from trauma. As much as we might like to plan, we have little control over random accidents, unforeseen acts of hostility, rampant viruses, or a stock market crash. Disruptions—minor irritations or major traumas—happen to everyone. Our responses and ability to recover from trauma are a measure of our health. Recovery is not about a return to the way things were, but adjusting as efficiently as possible to new circumstances and moving forward from there.

His second definition of health interlocks with the first. It is the ability to fulfill our avowed and unavowed dreams. A healthy person may live with great disabilities, or debilitating illnesses, yet still achieve more of their dreams than one living in dissatisfied comfort.

To achieve these definitions of health requires continuous learning and adaptability. The Feldenkrais Method is his framework for learning to be an adaptable, resilient human living in a world of ceaseless change. Moshe and every Feldenkrais practitioner since have worked with themselves and others toward self-reliance—to recover from trauma; and self-direction—to fulfil our dreams and put our intentions into actions at all levels of our lives.

The simplest exhortation embedded in his work is: "Don't get stuck"—move your attention, move your ideas, move your emotions, and move your body. Simply moving physically is not enough; the ability to learn and adapt through all aspects of yourself and your environment, with curiosity and discernment, are necessary companions.

Moshe Feldenkrais's own lessons were learned through challenges and injuries. Survival was never certain in his early years. Born in an Eastern European village intermittently ravaged by pogroms, he left his family at the age of fourteen and made his way overland to British Palestine. The ongoing lethal interactions between Arabs and Jews in his new country sparked a lifelong interest in martial arts. Largely self-educated, he worked his way to a place at the Sorbonne in Paris, where he achieved a doctorate in engineering. In Paris he worked as an engineer in the Curie laboratories, spending his leisure time as one of the first European students, then teachers, of judo. World War II ended this. Despite a badly damaged knee and his wife having a congenitally deformed hip, they limped to the coast and crossed to England. Once there, Moshe worked with the British Admiralty on sonar for submarines. Finally, in the 1950s he returned to Israel, working first for the Israeli government then for himself—developing a practice that would become the Feldenkrais Method.

By cultivating awareness through movement, people could break through cycles of self-defeating habits, he believed, and discover their highest potential as a dignified, potent human. The five books he wrote on his method are dense nuggets of wisdom for reaching physical, emotional, and intellectual potential.

Moshe Feldenkrais was noted for making the abstract concrete. He and others describing his work return to that phrase often. It is within this tradition that this book was conceived and written.

The TIYs are a strategy to convert the abstraction of reading into concrete experience. They are a shorthand form of a classic class structure in the Feldenkrais Method called "awareness through movement." These are verbally guided lessons that, like the TIYs, encourage students to investigate their own movement in more depth, using attention, discrimination, novelty, timing, repetition with variation—in fact all the processes of learning mentioned in this book. These processes build functional awareness that can be taken into any aspect of our daily lives. "Awareness through movement" lessons are designed to reacquaint students with the aesthetic pleasure of movement that we experienced as young children and can find again as adults.

With our clever brain's facility for abstraction, we can hide or skip details essential to achieving our potential. Reminding ourselves to return to the concrete, to the interwoven basics of learning and movement, is at the core of Feldenkrais's most deceptively simple, comforting maxim: "When you know what you do, you can do what you want."

Starting, Again

We began this book with five questions. Did you figure out the answers? Just in case you need it, here's where to find them in more detail.

HOW MIGHT A TIGHT TUMMY LEAD TO VOICE LOSS?

In OP4, Presence of Reversibility, we discussed Mei, the public speaker who was intermittently losing her voice. Combining video with sensory attention, she discovered a chain reaction that began with contracting her tummy:

When her face moved forward, her neck and throat tightened, and the sound became rougher.

As she became more skilled at noticing the extraneous contractions that led to hoarseness, she also noticed how much earlier the abdominal contractions happened with different audiences. Gradually Mei made a link between the anxiety she felt in front of small audiences and the increased work in her abdominal muscles.

Through exploring reversibility, she discovered resistance in the form of unnecessarily activated abdominal, neck, and chest muscles, which inhibited her freedom in breathing and speaking. By learning to sense and then reverse these involuntary contractions, she was able to free her voice and continue the work she loved.

WHAT DO SWINGING AN AXE AND A BABY'S FIRST MEANS OF PROPULSION HAVE IN COMMON?

In OP3, Homologous Movement, we described the powerful first means of propulsion a baby uses—sometimes called the frog hop or bunny hop. The same action developed in infancy remains in our repertoire for power:

In elite sports, this very early movement is used for rapid access to power. It gives us large forceful bursts, like the launching movement of the downhill skier or a swimmer off the starting block, the mighty downswing of the champion axeman, or the upward thrusting lifts of the Olympic weightlifter.

HOW CAN A BATHROOM SCALE TEST YOUR SKELETAL ALIGNMENT?

You explored this in TIY 2-2: Transfer Weight from Sitting to Standing (p. 46):

Transitions are the best way to test the effective alignment of the musculoskeletal system. Transitions require both local and global muscles to be working effectively in order to transmit force directly through the skeleton without damage or loss of energy.

An ideal use of the musculoskeletal system will show . . . a constant increase until you stand fully on the scale at your true weight without an overshoot. If you cannot do this, it will seem impossible . . . [but] it is a way of moving yourself that can be learned.

WHAT CAN WE LEARN FROM GIRAFFES ABOUT BALANCE?

In OP1, we used a photograph of a giraffe drinking to illustrate a more technical discussion about shifting loads and balancing objects:

As a giraffe lowers its great head and neck to the water, its center of gravity is moving down and significantly forward. The center of gravity is no longer over the standing base of support, so the giraffe must spread its front legs very wide and shift more weight into its back legs to prevent a survival-threatening nosedive.

We wanted also to show that you can learn from all sorts of teachers: from animals to painters, slack wire artists to babies . . .

AND—HOW CAN YOU USE THIS
INFORMATION TO LIVE A BETTER LIFE?

The simplest answer is: try it yourself. We have used the power of stories to illustrate the diverse applications and the surprising results that can emerge from a deeper acquaintance with these organizing principles. Apart from the foundation fable of the seven blind men and the elephant, all the stories are from Lesley's and Julie's lives and practices, practices of their colleagues, or from Moshe Feldenkrais's recorded work. Names and identifying details have been changed of course, but the essentials are intact.

One essential, common to all the stories, is their focus on "what" and "how": *what* someone was doing; *how* that impacted them; and *how* they changed.

The stories in our own lives tend to be "why" stories. *Why* we are like this, *why* we have made decisions, *why* we can or cannot do things. Science has found ample proof of our fallible memories and habitual misapplications of causality, yet we find the supposed certainty of our "why" stories comforting.

Exploring the seven organizing principles of movement gives each of us an opportunity to bypass the "why" and understand the "how" of what we do: *how* we take action, *how* we think, and *how* we feel.

We hope they will inspire you to keep exploring and expanding your ever-evolving potential.

REFERENCES

Alexander, Frederick M. *The Use of Self.* London: Orion, 2001. First published 1932.

Bly, Lois. *Motor Skill Acquisition in the First Year: An Illustrated Guide to Normal Development.* San Antonio, TX: Academic Press, 1998.

Bowman, Katy. *Move Your DNA: Restore Your Health Through Natural Movement.* Carlsborg, WA: Propriometrics, 2014.

Butler, David S., and G. Lorimer Moseley. *Explain Pain*, 2nd ed. Adelaide, Australia: NOI Group, 2013.

Claxton, Guy. *Wise Up: The Challenge of Lifelong Learning.* New York: Bloomsbury, 1999.

Doidge, Norman. *The Brain That Changes Itself: Stories of Personal Triumph from the Frontiers of Brain Science.* New York: Viking, 2007.

Feldenkrais, Moshe. *The Case of Nora: Body Awareness as Healing Therapy.* New York: Harper & Row, 1977.

———. *Awareness Through Movement: Health Exercises for Personal Growth.* San Francisco: Harper, 1990. First published 1972.

———. *The Elusive Obvious.* Cupertino, CA: Meta, 1981.

———. *The Master Moves.* Cupertino, CA: Meta, 1984.

———. *The Potent Self: A Study of Spontaneity and Compulsion.* Berkeley, CA: Frog Books/Somatic Resources, 2002. First published 1985.

Feldman Barrett, Lisa. *How Emotions Are Made: The Secret Life of the Brain.* Boston: Houghton Mifflin Harcourt, 2017.

Siegel, Daniel J. *Mindsight: Change Your Brain and Your Life.* Melbourne: Scribe, 2009.

Stukeley, William. *Memoirs of Sir Isaac Newton's Life.* 2004. First published 1752. Retrieved from The Newton Project: http://www.newtonproject.ox.ac.uk/view/texts/diplomatic/OTHE00001.

Thompson, Brad. *The Breathing Book: A Practical Guide to Natural Breathing.* Fitzroy, Australia: Red Dog, 2008.

Waitzkin, Joshua. *The Art of Learning: A Journey in the Pursuit of Excellence.* New York: Free Press, 2007.

INDEX

Italic page numbers indicate illustrations.

Feldenkrais Method, 14, 37,
172–174
Feldenkrais, Moshe, 172–174,
176
flexibility, loss off, 137–138
flexing/flexion muscles, 17–21,
18, 129
fear of falling, 29
homolateral movement, 50
forearms, alignment with hand
and wrist, 40–41, *41*
foreground sensations, 159–160
freedom of breath, 82–84
freeing the limbs, 129–132
using tools, 130–132,
130, 131
frog hop, 175
function vs. aesthetics, 124–125

G

Gates, Bill, 161
giraffes, 27, *28*, 42, 176
global muscles, 38
center and periphery working
together, 125
engaging for support, 136–137
gravity, 39, 41
releasing from support,
138–139
sitting rigidly, 124
strong muscles cover weakness,
136–138
transitions, 46
gravity, 121
jumping, 44
skeletal alignment, 39–42, *41*
Sir Isaac Newton, 2, 121, 124

gym workouts/weight training,
71–72, 74, 83–84, 124,
154–155

H

habit, non-habitual movement,
85–86, 163–164
Haeckel, Ernst, 49
hands, alignment with wrist, and
forearm, 40–41, *41*
head, 89–96, *90, 91*
lifting with attention, *123*
head and pelvis movement, 8,
87–89
head, 89–96, *90, 91*
pelvis, 102–116, *103, 104,
105, 110, 111, 113, 114,
115, 116*
rediscovering relationship of
parts to whole, 117
spine connection, 96–102,
98, 101
hips, 103–104
holding your breath, 82
homolateral movement, 50,
58–63, *60, 61, 62*
homologous movement, 50,
54–58, *55, 56*
How Emotions Are Made
(Barrett), 152

I

incompetence, embracing,
167–168
increasing resilience, 165–168
infants. *See* babies

ABOUT THE AUTHORS

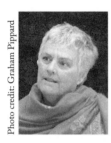

LESLEY MCLENNAN In 1983 Lesley was studying and performing mime in London, and struggling to achieve a particularly difficult balance sequence. Nothing really helped until the day she worked with Monika Pagneux, a diminutive, inquisitive woman, who invited Lesley to roll a smallish rubber ball under one foot for a couple of minutes and then recheck her balance. It was stunning. After the short, simple activity, Lesley easily achieved the complex balance. Moreover, when bending to touch her toes, her hand rested completely on the floor on that side, but on the "unworked" side only the fingertips reached the ground. How could two minutes rolling a ball under one foot stimulate balance, length, and flexibility? That was the afternoon Lesley got hooked on the wisdom that could bear such fruits. It represented such a completely different way of knowing the human body, and potentially of knowing about human beings.

Monika had been inspired by the work of Moshe Feldenkrais (more about this man and his method in OP7), and now Lesley was too. She trained as a practitioner and ran a part-time practice. Then, as often happens when life swirls us around, Lesley veered off into other arenas. Returning to practice after a long break and many detours, she found another fascinating teacher, very different from Monika but equally captivating in the depth and magic of her knowledge.

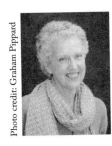

Photo credit: Graham Pippard

JULIE PECK had followed her curiosity from physiotherapy into a Feldenkrais training that changed the path of her professional and personal life. The ideas that are the foundation of this book come from Julie's exploration of her own physical challenges, her private practice, public teaching, studying source material, talking to colleagues, and some zillion hours of thoughtful action, broad reading, and deep reflection. Julie has worked with adults and infants, individuals with great talent, and others with most profound disability. As she adapted to increasingly diverse demands, she distilled more of her experiences into teachable chunks. Her life's work has been to uncover organizing principles of movement—those fundamentals that all babies must discover to grow into their potential and that all thinking adults can use to expand their potential.

This book is the result of a collaborative process. Lesley recognized in Julie's teaching a singular expression of underlying patterns in human movement. Julie trusted Lesley's curiosity and divergent thinking. Separating their voices and ideas would create more confusion than value, so in the book Julie and Lesley are "we."

About North Atlantic Books

North Atlantic Books (NAB) is an independent, nonprofit publisher committed to a bold exploration of the relationships between mind, body, spirit, and nature. Founded in 1974, NAB aims to nurture a holistic view of the arts, sciences, humanities, and healing. To make a donation or to learn more about our books, authors, events, and newsletter, please visit www.northatlanticbooks.com.

North Atlantic Books is the publishing arm of the Society for the Study of Native Arts and Sciences, a 501(c)(3) nonprofit educational organization that promotes cross-cultural perspectives linking scientific, social, and artistic fields. To learn how you can support us, please visit our website.